OH MY GOODNESS

IT HAPPENED TO

ME

MY JOURNEY WITH CANCER

JEAN A. LEACH

OH MY GOODNESS IT HAPPENED TO ME

About the Author

Jean Leach after suffering the trials and tribulations of living a life with cancer, decided to write a book to let all who might have to go through this ordeal, that they are not alone.

Her courage and strength gave her the outlook to just go on and fight this battle. She wanted to inspire others who are maybe going through the same kind of ordeal in life, to just keep going. Jean wanted to show people, that even though having cancer is a terrible thing to go through, there is always hope. To see the laughter in some situations that cannot be changed. She wanted people to take situations as they come and go on. Life is a very precious thing. Enjoy it, embrace it, live it.

I AM DEDICATING THIS BOOK TO ALL OF MY FAMILY AND FRIENDS WHO WERE THERE FOR ME DURING THIS TIME IN MY LIFE. I THANK THEM FOR ALL THEIR UNDERSTANDING, BUT MOST OF ALL FOR THEIR LOVE

Table of Contents

CHAPTER 1   DISCOVERY

As the words to a song go, " I don't remember what day it was, I don't remember what time it was", ring truth in my head, I think of the moment I felt the horrified feeling when I felt a lump in my breast. I felt fear, I felt uncertainty, I felt sorrow, I felt anger. The feelings swelled up in me like a wave of hot air rushing over my body. I was devastated and unprepared for the future to come. I guess no one ever is. You are never really ready to believe it is happening to you.

The question arose, "what do I do now"? I wondered to myself, was it really there or was I imagining it. I decided I better take control of the situation, and since I did not have appropriate insurance at the time, I would get to the local hospital clinic. I had a usual appointment for a few other things that ailed me at the time, and I spoke with a physician on the possibility of something being wrong. I also told him that I had felt a lump in my breast. I was seriously worried something could be wrong there also. He did an exam of the breast, and subsequently ordered a mammogram to be done. I know this is a normal thing to have done, but at that time I was frightened. The fear, the pain, and questions, take over your mind. The thought of the future outcome being uncertain, reigns in your mind. The thought of this one test could determine your future. The thought that you are putting your future in the life of a technologist and machine is unbearable.

The mammogram procedure is one that leaves you a little embarrassed, and a little sore, but cannot compare to the emotional feelings that are building up inside of you. What will the outcome be? Will everything be ok? Will the radiologist find something that is positively not what you want to see?

As you sit in that exam room waiting for the technologist to return to say you can get dressed, I feel, is the longest moment I can remember. I thought of how the films came out and how the nurse could not even give me a clue as to the outcome of the exam. You sit there and wait for what seems like a lifetime, in reality it is only a few minutes. You read a little, look around the waiting room a little, and daydream a little and think about the daily errands you will have to run. The waiting is just unbearable as your mind races through so many thoughts at once.

The nurse returns only to tell you "yes the films came out, but you will need to follow up with your physician for the results". At that moment, you know it will be another long wait. There is always an unending length of time you must endure until they make your appointment. It seems like that next appointment doesn't come soon enough. You're every waking hour, you think of how that one simple test can change your life. You think of all the possibilities. Maybe it will be negative, and everything will be fine, or will there be a question, and they might have to do more. And that ever lasting thought of the big "C" word that everyone fears, cancer. What will I do then? How will I tell my loved ones? Your days are filled with questions; your nights are filled with endless hours of tossing, and turning, and thinking.

Then the day finally arrives. Now is the doctor's appointment day. The day you learn your results. The day you get those results that you have waited so long to get. The day you learn if your future will change dramatically, or simply just go on. The day one physician can tell you what you have been questioning for so many days. A day you wish was over.

You go to the hospital clinic, and it seems like an endless wait. You sit in a room filled with people, wondering if they are awaiting the same information as you were. You wonder, how many women have already gotten their answers, and were awaiting a list of options? Your heart races, you feel like you are out of control. You know deep down in your soul, you have no ability to change this outcome. You have to trust in the radiologist who reads the films and the physician who gives the results. He is the physician that will give you his opinion and your options.

After what seems like a very long time sitting and waiting, you finally hear them call your name. The walk to the exam room, which is only a short distance, seems to be unbearably long now. My recollection of the nurse's words escapes me now. The moment was a moment of fear and anxiety. All I could think of was, the doctor will be in shortly, arriving to tell me my results of my mammogram. Something that has been building up inside of you for many days will now all be answered in just a moment. All the fears and all the anxieties will be answered. In a way you are glad that the day has finally come, but again you still fear the outcome.

People always say, "look at the bright side, it may be nothing". Yes, that is true, but in our inner being, the fear still exists, and is real. The fear of what the unknown will be. The inner feeling, that sense that you know something is wrong. I think every woman has an inner sense that tells you when something is wrong with your body. After all, you've had it your whole life! And you learn throughout your life how you positively should and should not feel. It's just a natural thing. We all know it, but we have to learn to listen to it.

As you sit in anticipation, you hear voices in the hallway. You hear nurses going from one room to another. You hear, "Please stand on the scale," "Please have a seat and the doctor will be with you shortly", "Please go to the front desk and they will schedule you a date for your surgery". All these sounds of the hustle and bustle of the never-ending line of patients ring in your ears. Each of those patients is awaiting their outcome. Each person is questioning his, or her "inner self". Each of those patients is awaiting answers to their questions. They are waiting for answers from one physician. One physician that can tell you if your life will be fine or tell you if your life will change forever. And for many of us it will change.

Sometimes the solution is simple; sometimes the solution is complicated and long term. But these physicians have the answers and we trust in their judgment. We are like little children, being guided by their parents. We all are waiting to be taken by the hand and shown the way to go. We put our trust in the physician's guidance for they have the answers. We do what we are told to do by the physicians, so that we may get over this occurrence in our lives and return to our every day lives as before.

As you sit and wait you hear the rustle of papers on the back of the exam room door. You know they are yours and the physician is reading the results. Those results you have been waiting for. Those are the results that hold your future. At that moment, you are filled with anxiety. As you sit, your heart pounds. You have to learn to just sit and breath deeply to get over this feeling. You think to yourself, it will be ok. Everything the physician will tell me will be just fine.

There is a knock on the door and you hear it open. You wait to see the physician's face. There will be the face of the man with the file. Can you tell by the physician's look? I don't think any of us can. I think every doctor is trained in medical school on how to smile when they enter a room. All the while they are holding your file in their hands. The file that holds the results you have been waiting for, and all you can see is this physician's smile. That one kind of smile that you know every patient has gotten every time the physician has entered his or her little exam room too. A conditioned smile I think at times, whether the tests are good or bad.

After that initial greeting, you wait for the physician to open that file, your file. The file that holds the contents that will decide your future. It is the file that has the information to change your life, or keep it the same. In my case, it seemed like an endless wait. He asked how I was feeling, and all I could think of was my inner-self saying opens the file. I cordially said, "ok", as most people do when asked that question. But inside, I felt like my heart wanted to jump out of my chest. There were butterflies in my stomach. Finally, I saw him open the file. The moment of truth had arrived. "Yes", he said, "we have gotten your results and there is a problem". It was a statement that I didn't want to hear. A statement none of us really believe we are going to hear. But then again, my inner-self had told me the same.

My heart sank at that moment. A feeling of despair took over the feeling of anticipation. There was that feeling of impending doom. The words rang in my head, for what seemed like forever. I remember not being able to say anything to the physician. I just waited there for the words I needed to hear to continue out of his mouth. He read the results to me, but they were more medical terminology then I could understand. All I could remember of that conversation was his words saying, "Yes, there was something that showed up in the mammogram and we need a biopsy". I was stunned. How could this be?

I remember him showing me the mammogram films and that wonderful little red circle that they put around the "suspicious spot", they are questioning. Those films stay in my mind forever. It was finally confirmed on those mammogram films, what my inner-self had been telling me all along. There was something wrong.

Now, was the question of what to do next? Physicians have a way of saying things in such a nonchalant way, that it seems like an ordinary thing. They are used to doing the same kind of thing day in and day out. Telling people what their results are. But I think to each and every one of us, it is not just an ordinary thing. It is happening to us and we are scared. To us, it is now our problem and we have to learn to accept it and deal with it. It is all so very hard to absorb in a short period of time. It is very hard to have a level head at this moment. Your mind is spinning and your thoughts are going wild with questions and wanting answers. But at this time, it is to your advantage to stay focused. It is a very hard thing to do. But you have to stay focused so you can understand what to do next. You have no idea as to what the next step is. After all this is the first time anything like this has happened to you.

As I sit there in that exam room, I remember hearing the words to other patients like "go to the front desk they will schedule your surgery". Now as I remember those words, the physician is repeating them to me. I could not believe this was happening to me. As physicians and patients do, you cordially say your goodbye's and head for the hallway.

Now the long walk down the hallway seems awfully short, because now all you can think of is those words the physician said, "we will need a biopsy". The procedure you know little about, the procedure that you are unsure of, the procedure that will tell you everything, and the procedure that will change your life forever.

Before you know it, you are there at the front desk and the nurse in front of you is calling for a date and time for your surgery. A date and time you really do fear in your heart. A date and time when you know the physician will find out exactly how bad or good things are. You won't know until it is over, until that next appointment, but you trust in the physician's abilities and schooling at this time. You are putting your trust in their hands.

You manage to stand there at the desk, what seems for endless moments, just so you can get your date and time and place for the surgery. You will get your date and time from a nurse that has so much going on at the same time, that the feelings of your own heartbreak is not even noticed. It is a normal thing for them to schedule surgery dates, over and over, and it seems like it is nothing more than they bat an eye at. They don't realize that this is the day that your life will change forever. Your life will never be the same. All the emotional feelings you were feeling when you came in to see the physician, were answered in a few minutes. But now this moment brings on more anxiety, more fears, more worries, and more questions.

You are once again like a small child. Just waiting for someone's guidance, someone's feeling of caring, someone's feeling of the fact that it will be ok. As you think of all these things, you stand there and wait for someone to say, "your date is", and to be at the hospital at this certain time. You stand in front of her like a lost child. No one can understand the feelings that sweep over you at this moment in time. Now you know the date and time is set. You know it has to be done, yet there are still more questions to be answered. As you stand before the nurse, your mind, and heart and soul, cannot believe this is happening to you. As you get ready to leave, you look at the nurse and say "thank you" as if it's a favor and you head towards the door.

Before you leave, you see a room filled with so many patients sitting, awaiting their turn. Some people are reading, some sleeping and some trying to control their children or keep them amused. They all seem ambivalent to whatever you have just been through. You know it is something that will change your life forever. You see their faces look at you as you walk out of that waiting room. It seems that they look at you to see what kind of expression you have on your face when you are leaving. Just like you might have done to someone else while you were waiting in that same room. Or maybe they are just thinking, "Oh, maybe now I will be next". Yes, they might be next to be learning their fate. They will be next to put their trust in the physician behind the door. They might be next to stand in front of that nurse who will schedule you to have something done that will change your life and your body forever. Learning that it will never be the same again. The thoughts and feelings in that waiting room are great. I guess no one ever really takes the time to notice that. I decided to just quietly walk out of the waiting room.

The walk to the car is one of thinking of the things that need to be done for this horrifying event. The pre-op exam, the blood tests, and all the things the hospital needs to know before you can have this procedure done. You get into your car and start the drive home. It seems you are not even thinking of where you are going, because the news that you have just been given, has consumed your thinking. You never think that it would happen to you, and when it does, your body and mind react to it in their own ways. You seem to put yourself on autopilot. Your body has a way of continuing on even when your mind is elsewhere. But fortunately you arrive at your destination safely; you are home. Now comes the next step to this whole ordeal. How do you figure out how to break the news to your family and friends? How do you tell them that your world has just fallen apart without upsetting them? That is the last thing you want to do at this point. You need family and friends to be your rock and upsetting them would not help. How do you break the news to them, and at the same time assure them that there is nothing to worry about. When at the same time, you are truly worried yourself.

I think all of us have that defensive mechanism that teaches us to just say, "it will be just fine". So you try to break it to your family and friends that "it's only a biopsy". There is nothing to worry about at this point. And it just needs to be done. You try to spare them the anxiety and worry that you are feeling right now. I think we all worry about how they will take it. Or maybe how will they handle the outcome? We always seem to put our own feelings aside and worry about how they will accept the news. It's only natural. We worry if they will be able to understand with the explanation I can only give them? I only hope I can give them an explanation that will give them a sense of assuredness that it will be ok.

My family is very understanding. All of them are, and so are my friends. My mother, "the saint of all good thoughts", always makes me feel better. She would say, " you should not worry about it, you can't do anything about it. Just have it done and wait and see". She said, "It will probably turn out fine". She knew in her heart how scared I was. Mother's can always tell that sort of thing without words even being spoken. That's what being a mother is all about. And being there when your children need you. Whether you are two years old or 40 years old.

Her advice was always good enough for me. She always gave me encouragement in my life, no matter what the problem may have been, big or small. She taught me always to have determination and she taught me how to love. She taught me how I could get through anything if I really wanted to. Just to rely on my inner self. She taught me how to be strong. My mother is my rock and always will be. My mother was my levelheaded leader. She always seemed to have the right answers to any question, whether it was about life, love, or just plain cooking! Mom was always there to listen, and believe me she is a wonderful listener. And boy could she give wonderful advice. Advice only a caring mother could give. I only hope that in life, I can give my daughter such advice like my mother gave me. And be able to lead her into the right direction and teach her determination and love.

So I took mom's advice and went on with my daily life. Even though I did, far back in my mind, there was still the fear and the anxiety. But I knew mom's advice and courage I could get through it. I knew she would want me to get up each day with the sun in my face, and go to work, and enjoy the day God had given to me. And so with that advice, I did. I tried my best to put it all in the back of my mind and go on.

Now, something you may not realize, while all this turmoil was going on in my life, I had a job that involved working with children of all ages for eight to sometimes 10 hours a day. Most days, my day was filled with the sound of laughter and children playing. Their day was just being happy to be able to come and play with friends. I loved to sit and give the children a blank piece of paper and tell them to make whatever they wanted to on it. These children could draw the world. Some of the wonderful things they drew you might not understand, but in their eyes it was something wonderful and they could tell you exactly what everything was on that paper and what it meant of course. These children, of all ages, races and whether they were boys or girls could put their emotions on those papers. They could put their fears on the paper, they could put their love on the paper, and they could put their happiness on the paper. They could do it with a simple mark of a crayon in their favorite color. One they picked out especially for each emotion. I saw life and love in these children. I saw happiness, I saw sorrow, I saw joy, and I saw anger. It seems funny how we do not take the time to realize that these little children are just like us grownups, just pint sized. They have feelings and thoughts and anxieties just like we do. They await your guidance just like we await the guidance of others. They put their trust in us, just as we put our trust in others. They look for that comforting thought, or gesture just as we do. Hopefully, they will find those things with ease.

Working with these children showed me how to enjoy life. They taught me how to take a moment of sorrow and change it into joy. They taught me that at a moment some problem seemed big, but in a moment's time, turned into something minor. And eventually, it was forgotten. These children taught me how to go home each day with a new outlook on life, something a child had to show me. That was something that I will always treasure. A single child can teach you many things, but a room full of children was fantastic.

I also used to watch two little girls when their mother and father "needed a night out". These little girls brought me so much happiness. I loved to spend time with them. We would have dinner, watch a little television, and of course, we would either color or play dress up. How wonderful playing dress up was. We used to dress up in the silliest of clothes and have a wonderful time using our imagination. We could be who ever we wanted to be and just have fun. We would be a princess or a witch or a fancy lady. Oh, and of course there was the ballerina, dancing around the living room to our heart's content.

Then when it was bedtime, I used to get to read them a book, which they had picked out. Oh how I loved that moment. There were the two little girls quietly awaiting just a small glimpse of fantasy. Something only books can give. It was something that a dream is made out of. Books were their favorite time. They used to get so excited. Those days made me so happy. Those two little girls brought joy into my life. And for that moment in time, I could forget all about what was going on in my life. I thank them for that.

Time went on and finally the day arrived for the procedure I had been dreading, and fearing. All the questions that had been going through my mind were there. What will it feel like? What will I look like afterwards? How big will the incision and impending scar be? And most of all, there is the worst question, what if they find cancer. All the questions and more go through your head as you wait. You sit in a registering room, waiting your turn to give your information to a person who sits at a desk taking information from dozens of people in a day. They are all waiting their turn. All waiting to put their trust in a physician they hardly know. All having to realize they are having surgery. This is the day. Surgery that will change their lives and the lives of their loved ones forever. Finally the registration process is over.

Then the moment arrives. The moment you have been waiting for. Finally, your name is called. At that moment you have a nurse take you to a room filled with other people behind curtains, having the same procedure, or other procedures done to them as will you. The nurse has you undress, put on a gown, and wait. The wonderful gowns they give you, the gowns that never seem to fit right, or just don't feel comfortable. It seems like time goes by so slowly. You wait patiently. Then the nurse finally comes back in to run the normal exam. They take your blood pressure, your temperature, anything they need to get started. Then there are the questions. The never-ending questions they ask. They try to make it as comfortable as possible for you. They try to reassure you that this is a normal line of questioning everyone gets asked to answer. We all have to answer.

Now is the time, where the nurse comes in that has to put in your intravenous needle into your vein. Will she use your arm or your hand? You cringe at the thought. Can she administer this without hurting you? Can she hit the vein the first time? Then she is finally ready with all of her supplies and she says at this point "you will feel a pinch". We all know the way we feel about that statement. I don't think that I have been pinched in a way that it feels anything like it does when that needle goes in. In a moment, if you are lucky, the procedure is over and done. They hook up a bag of fluid to the contraption attached to your vein, like it's a lifeline. You lay and watch the fluid drip, possibly wondering, "what if it stops"? You wonder, "what if there is a bubble in the line"? All those silly things and more that go through your mind as you lay and wait. It's quiet.

Then the nurse arrives again. This time she has some wonderful words for you. She asks, "Do you need to use the restroom"? You think to your self, "why didn't we do this before this lifeline got attached to my arm"? But like a little trooper, you figure you might as well try. After all, didn't your mother ever tell you "try to go before you leave"? Yes, we all know those words from our childhood and you figure that this is one of those moments that you should definitely listen to your mother's advice. How funny it is now, to think about those things when at that moment everything is totally serious. I guess that it is all the little bit of humor we all have inside of us.

So, the nurses try to get you up and walking without showing the world your naked behind. At the same time, you are trying to drag your attached lifeline with you. You are connected to tubes, in turn which are connected to a bag, which in turn is connected to a pole with wheels on it, which somehow you have to take along. What a chore that is to lug it all with you. And on top of it all, there has to be a trick to it. Hold the pole, hold your gown closed, and walk slowly not to get caught up in anything or slip.

So you make it to the restroom door and close it behind you. Ok, now what do you do? They don't give you instructions on going to the restroom, connected to all these wonderful things you have just dragged across the room. I think they should teach that as part of a course on getting a patient ready for surgery. Tips on how to maneuver your lifeline, while trying to use the restroom class 101. So, you manage to sit down, and then the time arrives that you will have to get back up. So you manage to lift yourself back up and decide to journey back to the bed. Again, slowly and carefully as not to fall, slip or pull anything out. You finally make it out of the restroom. As you look around for a nurse to help you back to your bed, you thank God for those funny little socks they give you with the grippers on the bottom. During this time, your mind is wondering, "what am I doing here"? Is this really happening to me? You have seen other people going through the same ordeal, but when it happens to you, it's all whole other story. You finally make it back to your bed as quickly as those sock covered feet can take you as not to show your behind. You get help from the nurse to get back into the bed, because we all know we don't have a clue as to how it's done in any simple manner. Now finally you are settled. The nurse goes on her merry way.

Now, the nurse comes back to tell you that an anesthesiologist will be with you shortly, to discuss the procedure for putting you to sleep. I don't know about anyone else, but the words "putting you to sleep" kind of worries me. Here is a specialist who can put you to sleep in a second, using his knowledge of chemistry and medications. Again, you are putting your trust into some one's hands. Again, the guidance and trust thing happens. Again, we await his words as to how he will do this "magic act", and what he will use. He tries to explain how they all work. You hear those words, the words we will have to trust in, "you won't feel a thing". Well, not until you feel that warm sensation going through your body. Then it is the feeling of you not being in control.

Now it is time to leave your life in their hands. To be left in the hands of all the doctors, the specialist and the nurses. That was the feeling I didn't like. I always like to feel that I am in control of my own body, and mind, and my own life. At that moment you are not.

Here come the smiling nurses ready to wheel you into the operating room. You talk to your loved ones, and bestow kisses before you leave. The vision you will see is of the ride going down the hall, and seeing the overhead lights go by one by one as you go. Then they reach the surgery room. By now your mind is so cluttered, you are thinking silly thoughts like "can they make it through that door without running into it"? Then there are those words "you'll feel a bump". I have no idea why that sticks in my head but it does. Do they mean a bump on the right, or a bump on the left, or a bump like a speed bump in the road? Your mind goes through so many changes at this time. You wonder about the surgery. You wonder how things are going to turn out. You wonder what they are going to do first when you enter the operating room. What will it be like? What will the nurses be doing? Will the doctor be in there right away to greet you? Will the anesthesiologist be ready to give you what you need to go to sleep during this whole ordeal, and will you wake up feeling fine or sick. At this time you end up in a room with nurses in gowns and masks running around busily. You wonder are they smiling under those masks? Or are they just going about their jobs like they do so many times a day. They count to three and a group of nurses lift you over to a table that is hard as a rock. The overhead light is so bright it blinds you. The room feels so cold. They offer you a blanket. They attach something to your finger, and strap your arm to a table. They let you know they are administering the anesthetic. Now you feel really out of control. No turning back now, even if you wanted to. You couldn't even lift a body part. You are now at their mercy. You trust that the surgeon will do his best to get everything out that he needs to. And without you even knowing it, times goes on. And the physician does his procedure as illustrated below.

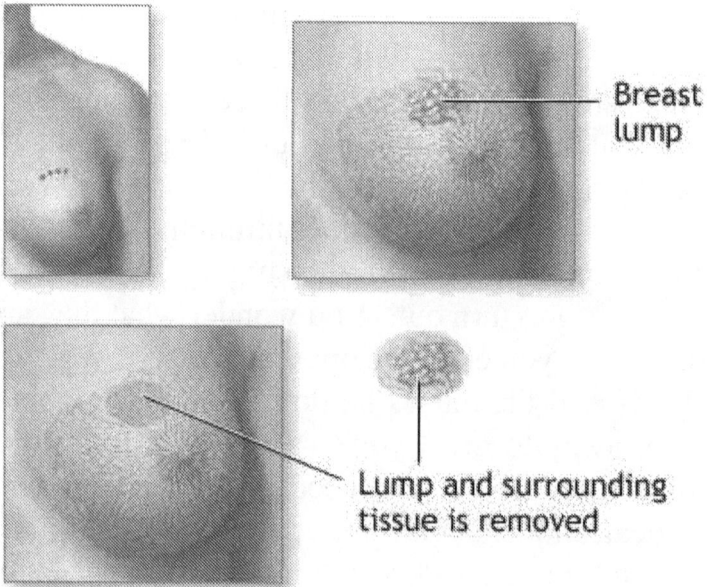

Breast lump

Lump and surrounding tissue is removed

OH MY GOODNESS IT HAPPENED TO ME

I remember awakening to the sound of someone's voice, saying "Jean wake up". Yes, easy for them to say I thought. Your eyes don't want to function and all you want to do is sleep. But now, and then, they arrive. So you decide to try and at least open your eyes. You open your eyes to view a room, again filled with people just like yourself who had no control of their actions either. We all are trying to wake up. We were all trying to wake up from a controlled sleep. We were all waiting to learn our fate, to know our future. We were all anxious to see what was done to our now transformed bodies from what they were before. To learn how they would never be the same again.

I think the first thing I tried to do when I had my thoughts in control was, to look under my gown to see if the breast was still there. The bandages were covering the incision, so I had no idea as to the size of the incision. That I thought will surely come in time. I just wanted to rest and thank God that the breast was still there.

Again, the nurse arrives. This time she is bringing you something to drink. You have to drink. We all know of course, you have to go to the restroom before they will let you go home no matter how good you feel. So it is really a must that you drink something even if you don't want to. Even though you drank all they have given you, you sit and wait patiently to have to go. I think that part of your body is slower to wake up, because it seems like forever. And now on top of everything you have a nurse coming over to your bed every 10 minutes or so asking you if you have to go to the restroom yet. It seems to be just like when you were a child and your parents were ready to go somewhere. They want you to go so badly before you leave and you have to convince yourself to go because they want you to. At this point it is only to make the nurse happy so you can go home.

Soon, you feel it's a good time to try or you will never go home. You call the nurse, and of course it is the same routine. It is a routine of trying to walk, holding your gown and towing your lifeline. On top of this all, you can feel your legs wanting to give out from beneath you. But you compose yourself, as we are all taught to do and give it a try. What a long way to that restroom it feels. Just standing up straight at this point in time is a task. You manage to arrive at your destination and close the door. But this time, you are at a disadvantage, because now you have had your surgery. No matter what part of your body you have had surgery on; it makes a difference when trying to use the restroom. Again, there are no instructions. We have to think of the easiest way of doing this task and we have to improvise. All the time sitting there, trying to convince yourself you have to go. By now you are feeling a little bit of pain, you are drowsy and you just want to lie down, but you know you have to do this, or not go home. Your mind takes over now and convinces your body to take over. Finally, thank goodness the task at hand is done and you know you can go home.

Now comes the trip back to the bed, which seems longer than the trip to the restroom. All the time, trying to hold your composure so you don't seem like a spectacle with you holding your gown and your lifeline. You finally make it to your bed and are allowed momentarily to rest. And at this point you need it.

Now, that you have done the task, a nurse arrives letting you know she will be bringing you some paperwork as if it was a prize for getting the job done. Again, you wait, but this time it is just fine because you welcome the break from all the activities expected of you. But as you rest, you think, "paperwork in my state of mind"? I don't think at this time I will remember a thing she says. Thank goodness it's on paper. At least later, when you have rested at home you can look over all she was telling you in those few moments. So you lay and wait for her to return with those glorious papers to sign.

While you are waiting, another nurse comes to take out the intravenous needle that has been implanted in your arm all the time. Again, you cringe at the thought. She gently pulls the tape holding it in off. Then suddenly without notice she pulls it out and it's over.

Now comes the nurse with the paperwork. I don't see how this is going to be feasible. She goes on to explain your limitations, your wound care, and everything they can think of to tell you at this time. Things don't register, as quickly when you are still not fully "there". So you listen and sign the papers when you are asked to.

Finally they give you your clothes back, which have been neatly put into a plastic bag. Now the hard part is getting dressed. But just like so many other events in your life, you manage. You know you will feel much better sitting there with your own clothes on. And you know the time is getting near when you will be able to go home to be with a family member, or your pets. Love needs to be with you when you get home. And it comes in many shapes and forms. But it's there. We just have to look for it.

CHAPTER 2   REALITY

As I sit at home, feeling the pain of the surgery, and wonder what the outcome may be, I think of all the things I have been through. There was the feeling of gladness that it was over with. Yet, there still was a feeling of fear, waiting for that next visit to the physician's office. Wondering how the pathology report came out. It always seems that the questions in your mind are endless. You have to learn to take control and get through the days to come.

As I take the time, to go and change the bandage on the incision, I see the part of me that will never be the same. I feel the anger at the thought that it had to happen to me in the first place. I took good care of myself. I ate good foods. What could I have done to deserve this happening to me? But I have to realize that there is nothing I can do about it now. The healing process is a difficult one. I take care of the incision as instructed by the nurses at the hospital. I take very good care of it, yet something is wrong. It was then, looking in the mirror, that I noticed a very large red area surrounding the incision site and was also moving slowly across the whole breast. Fear set in. There was fear of the unknown. No nurse can prepare you for something like this to happen. No instructions mentioned this happening. I knew it wasn't supposed to be this way. It was just not healing right. I called the physician's office and was informed it was just a normal situation and nothing to worry about. How can one answer such a question over the phone by not even looking at it? Again, I trusted them. So I just kept taking care of the site as I had been previously instructed to do. But as all of us do, we trust in our instincts. We trust to know how we are supposed to feel and know when something is just not right. It truly was not a good feeling I had. I knew deep inside that something was very wrong.

Thank goodness at this time, my daughter was staying with me. I was so very thankful just to have her near me for support and for her love. She helped take care of my wound even though it really made her ill to look at it. She really tried her hardest to help out with the bandage changing. My daughter is a very strong person. She, like myself, and my mother, are ones that can handle most situations and get through them. This one was very hard for her. This one involved her mother, which she had a hard time dealing with knowing I was in pain and worried that something was wrong. She never had to deal with anything like this before, but wanted with all her heart to help as much as she could. She's a wonderful daughter. She tried her best and did a wonderful job.

One day, while changing the bandage, we noticed something terribly wrong. She went to clean the wound, and the worst thing that could have happened did happen. When she went to touch my breast to clean it, a very large amount of a very ugly, horrible, disgusting, looking liquid came oozing out of the incision. My daughter immediately got ill. I felt so bad for her at that moment. I didn't care what was happening to me I felt bad for her for having to see it. I felt helpless to make her feel better. My heart sank at the thought of how she would remember this in her mind forever. It was something that affected me greatly and still does to this day. She, to this day can still remember that event vividly. She was hurt that it was hard for her to help me, and I in turn was hurt that I couldn't help her. The situation was upsetting for both of us, and will forever be in our memories.

Again, fearing the unknown, I called the physician and insisted on seeing him. Of course the usual wait ensued, even though I was oozing at the seems! I sit in the waiting room, again, waiting my turn. The room filled with people waiting their turn. Waiting for their results like I once did. Waiting there for just a little bit of reassurance that it will be all right. The faces of people not knowing what to expect or how to feel just like me all sat waiting.

I knew that I came to see the physician for the incision, but I also knew that in that little file in the door was the answer I had been waiting for. The results of the biopsy were in that file. I felt in a way, that I wanted to hear the results and yet a part of me did not out of fear. You try your hardest to think positive, but it isn't an easy thing to do. As usual, a nurse, who sits and takes down notes of your complaints for that day, lets you to a room. You sit and wonder does she really listen? Does she really understand your fear and anxiety? It seems like it's just another day for them in the clinic facility. I try to explain about the area overcoming my breast. I tried to explain the oozing liquid that came out of the incision. She just kept on writing, looked up at me and said, "the physician will be in shortly", and left the room. Well, thank you for your concern I thought to myself. In reality of things, at that moment, I was just another patient in a facility that was overcrowded with patients. In her eyes, I suppose she was worried about getting to the next patient.

Out in the hallway, you can hear that familiar sound of rustling papers on the door. You know that the physician is out there behind your door looking at your file. Now your heart begins to race. Your anxiety heightens. Then the door opens, and there is the physician with that smile. The conditioned smile I surmised. I remember sitting and trying to explain what was going on with the breast and the incision. He read the notes and finally decided to take a look. As he looked at the incision, he noticed that I was allergic to the tape they used for bandaging the wound. It literally too my skin off and left a very raw area where it was at. He decided to take all of it off. What a relief. I had no idea that I was allergic to that type of tape so I guess it was a good thing that I found out when I did.

The physician at this point looked at the incision. He informed me "oh it looks fine it's just healing". I knew that was not the case. I knew in my heart something was wrong. But as always we trust in what the physician with the schooling is telling us and we just take his word as being an educated decision. But at the same time, we have to realize that they are just human beings just like us. Just maybe a little more educated than the normal man on the street. Being in the position of wondering if it is healing right or not, I felt the physician should assess the situation and act on it accordingly. I felt this was not done. I felt robbed of treatment. As I sit there in despair trying to convey my fears, I feel my words are going right past him. Is he just in a hurry to get on with the next patient? Has it been a long day of patients, and I am just in there taking too long? As I sit there thinking, "this is useless", I see him reach for the file. That file will tell me what my future holds for me. That file will tell me if my world will change forever. As I see him rustle to find the paperwork, I wait. I only wish that he would hurry up and get it over with. As he reads over the results, I could see a change in his expression. He finally turns to me and says, "We have the pathology report". At this point, my heart is racing. It feels like I can't breathe. Then his next words rang out loud in my head. Please let it be ok I thought to myself. He had gone on about the pathology report verifying that it did come back positive for cancer. At this moment I was devastated. My head was spinning and I couldn't think straight. He went on to read the report to me, but it was so hard to understand. On the report are sentences and words us lay people just do not quite understand. All I heard was the word cancer.

At this point a fear came over me. What will I do now? What will happen next? What will happen to my breast? All this goes through your mind in a matter of seconds. And your worst fears buried deep inside of you are confirmed.

As he finishes reading the report, I said "what now"? He replied by saying "Well, we think we got it all so you won't need to do anything further". I remember those words very well. I thought to myself "we think we got it all". That was not very much assurance for me, but we believe. I was in shock. I was confused. As usual when going through a traumatic situation, you listen, you take the advice and believe in the physician that holds your life in his hands. At this point, I was relieved, and I was assured things would be fine, and I trusted in the physician who made the decision. After all, he was the physician with the schooling.

I left his office with relief, not having to stop at that desk for more appointments. After all, the physician was the one with all the knowledge, all the answers, and the once to make all the decisions. I kept telling myself that over and over. I trusted him. So, you go about your daily activities. Thinking everything will be fine. You inform your family and friends that the physician said it will be fine. You feel good that you can give them this bit of information. Your day is filled with content and relief and so, as usual, life goes on.

CHAPTER 3   LIFE GOES ON

Throughout the following weeks the healing took place. There was not only physical healing but also emotional healing as well. It was hard to deal with all the feelings that have been going on with myself and my family and friends. I had a hard time dealing with the emotional feelings of my daughter. I know she was scared. I know she was worried. I am very close to her and I hope in my heart she will never have to go through the same thing I have gone through. I hope that she never has to find a lump in her breast or anywhere else for that matter. I hope that she never has to feel the anxiety of waiting and not knowing. I hope she never has to have the stress of going for tests, and waiting for answers. I know that she fears that some-day, I would not make it if this ever happened again in some other part of my body. It hurt me inside to know that my daughter had to live with this feeling of the uncertainty of how long I would be with her and the family.

When you go through something like this, something that is so devastating and so traumatic in our lives, the questions always seem to sneak into our every day lives also. I too, had that fear, the fear of how long I will be with my loved ones. What will the future be like? But as usual, the physician as-sured me that things would be just fine. I would need no fur-ther treatment. They think they had gotten it all.

As the days went on and the healing continued, I felt something was wrong. It was just not the way it should be.

There was a very large blood spot completely going across my breast area. It scared me, but as before I was assured that everything was ok. The incision eventually closed completely. Eventually the large blood spot eased up also. To this day I still do not have an answer as to what that was.

Throughout this whole experience with the breast, I also had some abdominal pain. At this point, your mind plays tricks and suggests to you maybe something is wrong there too?

At this point, I finally got good enough insurance that I could go to a facility that took my kind of insurance. I decided I needed a regular physician for regular needs not only how I was feeling at this point. I wanted to feel that this would be a physician that I could trust. I felt that if I could go to a female physician she might be able to understand my feelings and fears about this cancer episode a little bit better. So, I gathered up my emotions, and fears, and questions, and called a female physician's office for an appointment in a very well known facility. In my heart, I thought, "this is it", I will find someone who will be able to understand everything that I have been feeling and fearing. This woman physician would be able to listen to my complaints like they were real and not just my imagination. I know how I felt. I knew it still was bothering me and tender. It was time to find another physician who would give me an answer as to what was going on with the breast at this point.

I made an appointment with the woman physician's office, and trudged to the hospital like a good little soldier going into battle to fight the never-ending foe. I put trust in my decision, knowing that this place will know what to do. It was a large facility and someone there would be able to help.

I sat in the waiting room, thinking of how I did this so many times before, elsewhere, waiting. This was a very nice place, and I thought there would be very qualified physicians working there. My fears seemed a little more relieved. It was a beautiful place, many nurses, and people going in and out at regular intervals. They were all hoping that their visit would be a good one. I was anxious to tell this woman physician all about my anxieties pains and worries. I thought she would be the one to understand. I was hoping she would be the physician that would ease my mind and tell me what to do.

I sat along with everyone else in that waiting room, anxiously waiting my turn to see the physician. Then I heard my name being called. It seemed like a very busy office, nurses running all over, doing whatever it is they needed to do, ambivalent to what was going on elsewhere. A nurse had me follow her and showed me into a room. She took the usual data, blood pressure, heart rate, temperature, and weight. She sat down at the small writing area and started asking me questions. Now these questions are geared to every person coming into this room. Then came the question, "what are you here for today"? I tried my best to explain the situation I had just been in. I tried to explain the traumatic finding of cancer, and the question of no treatment after surgery. I told her I felt something was not right with the breast. I also talked with her about the abdominal pain I was experiencing. The nurse continued to write in the space allowed for comments to be seen by the physician. After the previous physician's uncaring attitude, I was worried about every word put down. The nurse finished writing, and the well-known words took their place in that little room, "the doctor will be in with you shortly". Oh, how those words ring in your head. You sit and think of all the things you would like to mention to the physician. You think of all the things that have been going on in your mind since you made the decision to call for this appointment. How funny it is, that our mind can go through so many thoughts in a matter of quick minutes, while it seems like an endless number of minutes waiting. At that time you are just waiting for that knock on the door you so long waited for.

Then the knock, and in walks the physician you are trusting with your life once again. As the physician enters, there is that smile. Is it a real smile or the one they maybe teach in medical school? After the initial greeting, she goes about her business of reading what the nurse had entered into the file.

As I sat there, I wondered if this physician is the physician that can answer my questions? She doesn't seem to be very personable. Again, my heart questioned am I doing the right thing. I was getting an uneasy feeling. And again, there is my inner self talking to me again. Is this whom I want? This woman physician seems very professional and it will all be fine. I sat and waited for her to finish reading the chart notes. She looked up from the notes and said to me, "and what brings you here today"?

Well, in my mind, I thought, "didn't the nurse just write that down and didn't you just read all the information"? But as usual, you put your trust in the physician and you just go ahead and repeat everything you just told the nurse five minutes before. It would be everything that is already written down in those notes or so we hope. I didn't get a close feeling with this woman physician that I was hoping for. I went on to tell her about the previous problems and the cancer. I told her about the pains I was having in the breast. The feeling of closeness never came. The feeling of understanding and compassion never came. It was like being in a room with a machine. It was like she was a machine that really was programmed, to take information and formulate an answer from that information. It was all kind of mechanical and sad. I thought to myself, did this woman physician have no feelings?

I even went through the normal procedure of putting on the gown for the examination. Of course at this time, the physician left the room to go do, what ever it is they do while they are waiting for you to change. I think they see the next patient to save time during their day then go back to you.

Then the door opened again, and the examination went on. While she was examining me, I tried to explain the fears and thoughts of my cancer diagnosis. I tried to explain the feeling that maybe something else should be done because there was still pain. I tried to explain the abdominal pain also, which was an issue at that time. And again, the exam went on with no comment or regard for what I was saying. Wouldn't things go much easier if physicians would just listen to what you are saying? She geared herself more to the abdominal pain then the breast issue I told her about. I guess I felt she figured it was not important, because the other physician said it would be ok and that was good enough for her not to worry about it. I felt like she was thinking that I was just another complaining patient. But I wanted her to listen to what I had to say about the breast. She decided to do tests. Routine tests. I tried again to tell her about the breast pain, and again I was partially ignored. She had said, "Oh it's just healing, everything should be fine". She decided to do a mammogram in a few months. But I was worried now. I just couldn't convey the importance of my worries about this whole experience to this woman physician. You would think that being a woman physician she would be a little more caring and do a little more in depth testing or send me to someone else for an opinion. She did not. Again, we have to put our trust in a physician who should know the steps to take. I didn't want to wait a few months; I wanted answers now while the pain was there. I wanted her to listen now. But we trust in them and I waited. I thought about her decision and hoped that she knew exactly what I needed at that time because the decision that she made could affect the rest of my life, and it did.

I went on with my life as usual, always wondering if she did the right thing, but again trusted in her ability. Through subsequent visits, the breast issue was not addressed again. We all know when something is wrong with our bodies. We ask ourselves, "Is it all in my mind, because no one seems to listen or be worried but me". But I knew there was something that was just not right in the breast. It was just not how it should be feeling. But again, we trust in our physician.

CHAPTER 4   DECISIONS

As time went by, and many visits later, I learned I needed to find a better physician. I was just not satisfied. I knew deep inside that something was not right. The female physician I had hoped to trust and confide in for a solution was not helping in any way. It seemed that she just was not listening.

I decided to go beyond my present situation, since I was being ignored as to my complaints expressed. Now, not only was their pain in my abdomen, but also my breast incision was still hurting and sore. This was an ongoing development that I was afraid of.

I decided to take my life in my own hands again. I needed to gain control of the situation. Since I still had the abdominal pain, "female problems" I presumed, I called and made an appointment with a gynecologist at the same facility. I was nervous, I was scared, but my inner self said, "Try again". Someone had to listen I thought. Someone had to care.

I had to wait for an appointment of course. This took time and days turned into weeks until I could see another physician. This was another female physician. I was hoping that this one would listen.

I arrived at the appointment anxious, fearful but oh so ready. I was determined that this physician would listen.

God must have heard me when I asked for direction. As I walked to the building where the gynecologist was, it was beautiful. Nurses and workers that I passed by were saying "hello", that had never seen me before. This was a pleasing scenario. I was pleased. For once, I felt inside, that I was guided to the right place.

As I entered the elevator to go to another floor, as those doors closed, my heartbeat was increasing. You wonder what you will see when those doors open. Would it be a warm and inviting place or a cold orderly robotic place?

Soon, there was my floor. The elevator stopped and the doors opened. There, to my satisfaction, was a beautiful waiting area, with lots of room and lots of chairs. Over in the other area, there was the receptionist, who took your information and the nurses that called the patients.

I walked slowly over to the receptionist's desk like a child going to the front of the class. I felt like all eyes were on me. There were actually happy people, sitting waiting their turn. Wondering in silence what they thought you were there for. All sitting waiting for their name to be called, to give information to get a physical or just to hear their fate whether good or bad.

As I stood there, I could hear a nurse saying those words that rang in my every being, "we'll set up your surgery time and date". How I remember those words being said to me and here there was someone else hearing those very words. My heart went out to them. But in this case, the nurse was actually saying it with some compassion. She cared. She knew how that person was feeling. She actually tried to make this patient feel comfortable and not so afraid. How nice that was to see.

I noticed in the area, an abundance of workers doing their assigned job descriptions, but all with a smile and a true sense of caring. It truly was a pleasant surprise. One of the workers looked up and in a pleasant comforting voice said, "Can I help you?" I said, "Yes I have an appointment." She asked that I fill out the usual forms, and for copies of my insurance. But yet, they were very pleasant in the way they approached you asking for what they needed. She finished what she had to do and informed me that I could have a seat and someone would be with me. It was a pleasant experience.

I sat down in the waiting room and admired the paintings on the walls and the beautiful wall of windows to let the sunshine in. What a wonderful way to wait, with art and nature. At this moment I began to relax. Maybe this will work out I thought to myself. Maybe this is what I have been looking for.

As I sat quietly, I heard my name called. As I looked up, I saw a very pleasant woman in nurse's uniform waiting for me. I walked towards her only to notice the smile on her face was actually, genuinely, honest. And that was a wonderful feeling. That is what makes a difference in how you feel.

We said our hellos and walked down the hall. Then, without hesitation, came those wonderful words we all dread. She said, "can you step on the scale so we can get your weight"? Now as I see it, we all secretly know how much we weigh. We all have taken the time to check at home in the morning of course, how much we weigh and maybe to check the accuracy of our home scales. We stand there and wonder, will they take off a pound for me shoes? Oh and my clothes have to account for two more pounds at least! Soon it's over and it's either a good surprise or a bad one. Or, maybe their scale is just off? Maybe it was that extra cup of coffee in the morning that did it. I will have to try and remember that.

So, you both continue down the hall to your assigned room. I was thinking to myself, would this nurse actually listen? Will she hear my complaints or just write the "important to her" remarks. To my surprise, she was wonderful. She explained the "first time" procedures and took the normal blood pressure, temp readings etc. Now for me, the test would begin. The notes. Those notes that could make your visit, or break your visit. Would she really write down what you were saying or what she felt should be written down for the doctor to view. Her vision of your complaints put down in her writing.

She started out by letting me speak my mind, and she would listen and take notes and she actually did just that. If something I said concerned her, she would ask a few questions and write more. I was so pleased at her professionalism and yet her sense of true concern. Again, it was wonderful.

It seemed like we talked for an hour but truly was only a few moments in time. She said, "now that this is done, lets get you a gown and I'll go get the physician". It was done so pleasantly, that you really didn't mind the gowns that opened up in the front this time bearing your all to whomever enters what space is now yours.

Then there is that waiting period we all dread. The time you have to spend alone in that room waiting for the physician to come in. You are always anxious it seems. By now, you have read all the charts on the wall, and you know every part of the human reproductive organs, since you are in a room that is designed for just that.

Then you hear the lifting of the chart from the door. Now again, your heart begins to race. Are they really reading the notes the nurse has made, or just getting your name and statistics?

The door slowly opened, and to my surprise a very pretty, young, perfect smiling physician appeared. It wasn't the normal medical school smile. This one was genuine. She called me by my name when speaking to me, and said how nice it was to meet me. She shook my hand with professionalism but yet with compassion for how I must have been feeling.

Then, to my surprise, she said she had read the notes and wanted to examine me further. She actually read the notes.

What a wonderful feeling that was. No repeating every detail I just went over with the nurse.

The exam was the normal gynecological exam, except for one difference. She did truly care. She took her time to know my feelings and fears all the time she did her work. It made me feel trusting, something I hadn't felt in a very long time. We talked about the abdominal pain and the breast pain.

At this point, she was shocked and surprised, that no further treatment was given after the first breast cancer surgery. It seemed that radiation or chemotherapy was in question. She was truly worried about the breast because it was still painful on the incision site. She assured me that she would consult a few other doctors she knew and get back to me on it. I truly trusted her. I knew she was the right choice for me.

Since I was also having abdominal, problems female reproductive problems at the time, we centered on those problems. Tests, medications, anything she thought I needed for those symptoms, but she never gave up finding an answer to the breast problem. She always took time to listen and care.

As the days and weeks went on, my female problems took president over the breast question. In her eyes, I still needed a primary care physician. We talked about the physician; the female one, that I had tried before and I told her I would never go back to her. She said her nurses had a list of physicians who could be just that someone for normal checkups, or to authorize any surgery to be done if I needed it in the future.

The physician's nurse set up the normal return dates, with smiles and accommodating efforts. Then someone else picked a name of a doctor who I could use for the small things, a regular family physician. I agreed since in my eyes, it was a pick out of the hat situation. I figured how bad could this be it's just for checkups.

So, I left this new physician's office with a sense of peace. She listened, she took care of my problem, and assured me we will continue on track with the breast situation. I agreed. At this moment I felt relieved.

Now the day came when I would see the "other" physician for the purpose of setting up primary care physician. The day came, the time came, and the receptionist at this physician's office seemed to feel the same way. As if it was just another day. Sad I thought to myself. I was hoping that this was not an indication of "this" doctor's attitude. But it was.

I went through the normal procedures of registration, and also giving the nurse the information she needed for the notes in the chart. At this time I had to add a sore foot to the list of pains. Somehow, I managed to hurt it, where and when I do not remember.

As the physician entered the room, I was greeted with a smile and also the statement, "I know you are here for the purpose of setting up a primary care physician and a check up, but I can't be that physician, I am going into another field of specialty at this facility. But I will see you today". My heart sank. Why did they even send me here? I was confused. But I guess the nurses who made the appointment with him were not informed of his plans.

Well, again to my surprise, after reading my history of cancer and looking at my foot, he said, "your foot is a little blue but it will be fine, and also you are just plain overweight". He reached for a piece of paper with a diet on it and left the room. To say the least, I cried all the way home. It was horrible. I was totally devastated and hurt. I just didn't know how to take anymore.

Weeks went by and my abdominal pains got worse. I was hemorrhaging badly. I called the gynecologist, who I knew would help immediately. She had me come into her office right away. I was scared and she was very, very comforting. It was so bad of a situation, that she scheduled a hysterectomy right away. She also informed me she had spoken to a surgeon there at the facility, and that he was anxious to see me about my breast problems. I was scared but thrilled at hearing this news as it still was bothering me. It eased my mind. She also arranged for me to see an oncologist at that same facility. Maybe he could give some insight as to why nothing was done after the breast surgery in the past.

I had the hysterectomy in Dec. of 2000. It went well, and no problems. My gynecologist was the most wonderful physician I could ever ask for. There was always a kind word, or a phone call to see how I was doing. As the weeks went by and I healed, I saw the oncologist at the same facility. He was a wonderful caring person also. During my visit he was amazed that I had no radiation or chemotherapy after the first sign of cancer breast surgery. When he realized there was still pain, I was sent to the surgeon that my gynecologist recommended.

The surgeon was surprised to see me back. He thought they would have started radiation. But when he learned that the oncologist sent me back because there was pain at the old incision site, he then too was concerned.

Again, the series of events started. There was testing, discussions, doctor visit, and biopsy. I couldn't believe I was going through it all again. But this time I knew I was in good hands. Not like before and that really helped ease the anxiety.

Well the day came when I would have to go in to get my results again. The difference now was that I knew deep down what it was. I had a feeling that the cancer had returned.

As I sat in my new surgeon's office I could feel that fear, and anxiety I felt so many times before. Again, I waited for that door to open. It eventually did. By the look on the surgeon's face, my fears multiplied. My gut feelings were "oh no not again". He tried to break it to me gently, but the news still stabbed me like a knife, at my heart and soul. Yes, it was back, the cancer was back, and in the same place it was before. "How can that be?" I thought. But it was true. Now what to do was the question.

As I sat there listening to the physician speak, his words seemed endless. His words seemed like I wasn't really hearing them but I was. Yes, they found more cancer, now what to do was the question. I heard him speaking as if it was in a dream. All I heard was the word mastectomy. My heart sank, my body started to shake from the shock. I couldn't believe what I was hearing. How can this happen in such a short time. How can it come back in the same area? I was hurt and confused. My surgeon tried the best he could to explain, but it didn't help the devastation. I suppose he realized my present state of mind, and decided it would be best to talk again later. He offered counseling, which at the time I couldn't even think about. He said he would like to have a conversation with both the oncologist that saw me previously and a plastic surgeon they had at the facility. He thought I would have a good chance at having what was called a tram flap. You see, I guess my body which was shaped in a way like a kangaroo's pouch, made me a perfect candidate for this type of surgery and I would look as good as new. At least he tried to make me feel that way. It did help in a way.

The drive home was so very long. My road to home was a very large, highly traveled highway. Most of the way home, I was in shock. How could this happen. The previous surgeon who did the surgery said I did not need any more treatment and everything would be fine. Well, it's not ok I thought to myself as I drove. I went at that moment from being into shock to being full of anger. Why, was the question? Why wasn't anything done before to alleviate the possibility of this happening. My mind filled with questions about what would happen now. Will I be scarred for life, emotionally and physically? I answered my own question at that point; "yes it would".

Somehow, under God's guidance, I made it home safely. I entered my home, gave the dog's kisses and hugs and cried myself to sleep. When I awoke, I realized my Labrador dog Stormy, never left my side. She knew something was wrong. She sensed she needed to be close. For that moment, she was my rock and my sanity. She loved me for me, and knew I was hurting. I wonder how animals can sense that, but I truly believe that they can. I know she did. From that day on, she was always by my side, day and night. She knew. And she always wanted to comfort me. She sensed my anxiety and fear. I really needed her that day and she was there for me. She was truly my loving pet. She did love me no matter what, and I loved her.

CHAPTER 5   NEW HORIZONS

As the days and weeks went by, with the anticipation of the future medical surgery and treatments, my anxiety grew. I waited patiently for my surgeon's call on how he and the plastic surgeon and oncologist would proceed. I spent every spare moment looking up the procedure on the Internet and knew I would be informed, not like the last surgery. I looked at what was going to happen to me. It frightened me, but I knew if I researched it all, it wouldn't leave me with such a shock as to what I would look like and how I would feel. It wasn't a pretty sight. But I knew I had to deal with what was going to happen and get through it. The days went by filled with anticipation and apprehension.

Then the phone call came. My surgeon informed me between all the doctors, this would be the best option for me, and he would have his nurse talk to the plastic surgeon's office for an appointment, and to schedule a time for both of them to be in the operating room. I thought this was wonderful for everyone to be communicating. It eased my mind.

You see, as the surgery goes, the first doctor would remove the original cancerous breast, and the plastic surgeon would then come in and rebuild it. It was going to be a very, very long surgery. All I could say to him at that time was "ok, let me know". You are in such shock that you just agree.

OH MY GOODNESS IT HAPPENED TO ME

I received a call from my surgeon's office. The nurse calmly, but apathetically said, "This is the name of your plastic surgeon at our facility, and this is your appointment time". Again, all I could say was "thank you". My regular surgeon's office was very compassionate as to how you feel. I thought o myself how wonderful it was to have a surgeon who is not only professional, but also caring. It was a relief I needed to have. I finally had trust in someone. What a wonderful feeling it was. My fears didn't seem so bad.

The day came when I was to have my appointment with my plastic surgeon. As I drove to his office, I didn't feel the anxiety I felt before. I just knew it would be just fine. This surgeon can make me whole again. He will help me get through this. I can actually look normal again.

His office was a beautiful one. Nice surroundings, nice people, very busy office. I sat calmly and waited for my name to be called. I saw many people with bandages from plastic surgeries. Hands, legs, faces, I wondered if they were accidents, or just wanted the work to be done. I hear no complaints as I waited in that room. No grumping about waiting too long, or not getting the right care. Again, it was wonderful.

Finally, my name was called. I got kind of nervous at this point. I went with a nurse, who directed me to an exam room. She took the necessary information, and also informed me that they had my information on my circumstances from my regular surgeon. This was a surprise to me. The two surgeons had not only talked, but also shared information about me. When I thought I was just another patient, I was actually a concern for them both. Again this was wonderful and promising.

The nurse left and I waited for the plastic surgeon to come in. Appropriately awaiting his arrival with the typical open front paper gown. It seems you always try to keep it closed, not just for modesty, but also for warmth. The rooms always seem so cold. I had never been to a plastic surgeon before for anything. I wondered what it would be like especially for what I was there for. Would he be able to make this all better and make me whole and new?

I could hear the rustle of paper on the door. I heard a knock and I said, "Come in". A very nice gentleman entered the room with an outstretched hand and introduced himself. How nice that was. That little "for real", kind of gesture he gave really did mean a lot to me.

He went on to explain how he knew the background of my case, and would like to do an exam to see if I would be a good candidate for the tram flap type of surgery he and my surgeon spoke about. I was fine with that, considering how many doctors saw my naked body already. The feeling of embarrassment was "old hat" by now. So I thought.

The next thing kind of came unexpectedly. He said, "I'll need to take some pictures for the file". I thought to myself, "How strange is that"? But I guess it was a routine procedure in an office of this type. He went on to inform me that a nurse would be present also. I thought to myself, "Oh boy, another person there looking at me". But inside it kind of made me laugh to think such things.

Now I ask you, how weird and uncomfortable can it get to stand there with an open front gown, having a person you never saw before in your life take photos of your breasts and abdomen? I guess for some woman, having that happen, in a non-physician scenario would be ok, but for me it seemed very strange and uncomfortable. They did their best to make me feel like it was nothing but routine. After all, he was taking pictures of a scarred up breast and an abdomen that looked like a kangaroo's pouch! After it was over, I laughed at myself for having to even think about it. How silly that was. But this was a whole new experience for me, one I was not prepared for. It was a situation that will always seem comical to me.

Then came the physical examination. The breast was very sore to the touch, so it was a very painful exam, but necessary. I had just had the hysterectomy shortly before the Appointment so the abdomen was tender also. But it all went smoothly and quickly, which was wonderful for me. He was a very caring and sympathetic physician.

He went on to inform me how I would be a good candidate for a tram flap, and tried to fill me in on the procedures of such a tremendous operation, and how good it would be to have my own live tissue forming the new breast and get a tummy tuck too. How great I thought. He actually made me feel like this whole ordeal will be a good thing. That was a nice feeling. The long surgery time kind of worried me, but for a surgery like this it was normal.

The surgery to me was going to go like this. They take the original breast off, leaving the skin. Then they make a cut in your lower abdomen and cut a large portion of your muscle but not completely out. It is just rerouted up your chest to form the breast with living tissue and original arteries and veins flowing. Hopefully, keeping it all alive. It really did make sense to me at the time. It seemed a very tedious and time consuming surgery, but one that was explained to me very clearly. Which really did help. And so I agreed to what they wanted to do. It seemed like it was a good idea and healthier for me. It had to be done in any case I might as well do it the way that will come out the best in their eyes. The procedure is shown in the following illustration. To me this was the best way to have this surgery done. All in all I think my plastic surgeon made a very good decision on how this type of surgery should be done because of the shape of my body.

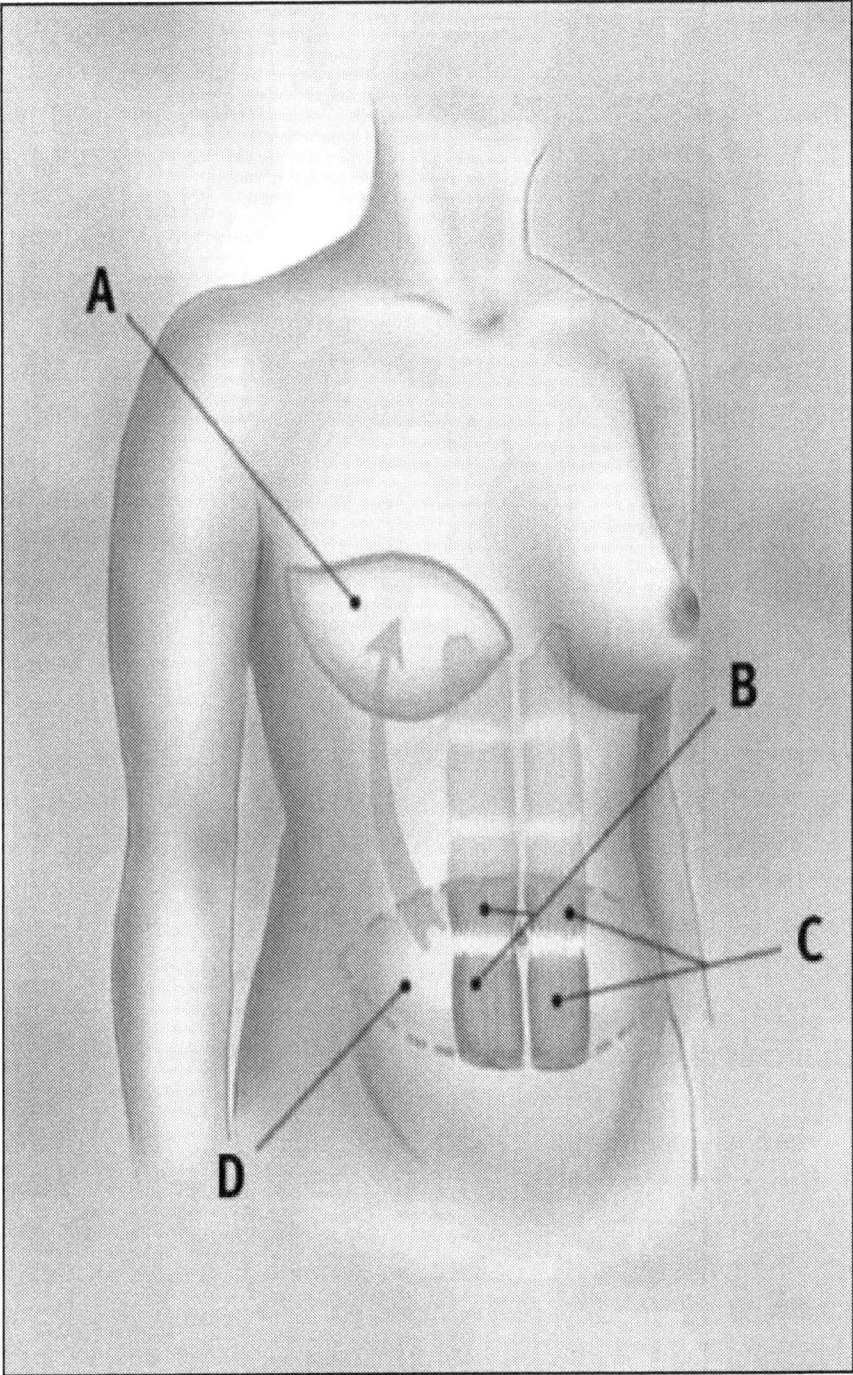

I decided to leave the technical things to the surgeons. Unfortunately, there were a few obstacles we had to overcome though. For one, I was allergic to most antibiotics, and second to morphine, which is the painkiller "most often prescribed", for this type of surgery. We had found this out when I had my hysterectomy previously. My eyes swelled up from that particular pain killing medication. But I knew no matter how painful it will be I would have to get through this if I wanted a new lease on life. And I did want that. I wanted to be beautiful again and whole again. And most of all, I wanted to be cancer free.

This time I went home with a feeling of ease. Now knowing the professionalism of the plastic surgeon helped. Every little detail was explained to me. Including the fact that there would be subsequent days of intensive care after the surgery. Being the headstrong person that I am I knew that I could get through this.

In my wildest dreams, and even with all the research I did on the procedure, I could not have been prepared enough for what was about to happen. It would change my life and my looks forever. I would never be the same physically again. Because of this cancer, I would never be the person I was before. I would never be able to look at myself in the mirror again without thinking of all that has happened to me. I would be thinking every day from then on would the cancer return again?

But as I mentioned, I had complete trust in my surgeon and plastic surgeon, something I didn't have before now. Deep down inside I knew they would do their best to make me somewhat what I was like before. Whenever you have surgery, you are scarred in a new place, never to be the same. It takes a toll on your heart, soul, and mind. It engulfs your days and nights. A part of your life is changed forever. Now is the time when you will just have to accept it and move on. Easier said than done.

CHAPTER 6   THE DAY HAS ARRIVED

Days went by with the usual trips to the hospital for everything that you might need before the surgery date. I had to do all the blood work, electrocardiogram, chest x-ray if needed, and insurance numbers.

After all the preadmission testing was completed, I waited for the day of the surgery to arrive. I was very anxious, not only for the day to arrive, but thinking of the outcome and how it would look and would everything turn out fine. I think those days are the hardest, you are constantly thinking of how things will go during and after surgery.

At this time I was fortunate enough to have a Personal Assisting position that I could work out of my home. My employer was very understanding. He bought me a computer for my apartment, and storage units for my files. It helped keep me very busy dealing with financial matters because it commanded my utmost attention. It helped keep my mind focused and my sanity. I welcomed the time to be kept very busy.

As the surgery day got closer, my mind wondered in many directions. I knew it would be a very rough road of recuperation. A long road of healing physically and mentally from something I couldn't control. I planned my days so that after surgery, it would be easy to recuperate. I planned daily tasks and meals that would be healthy for me. The family that I babysat for were wonderful. They offered to help me in any way possible. They even made little meals for me to eat while I was recuperating. They were all put in little containers to heat up when I wished to eat. They had all kinds of other little things in that package just to make me feel better. It was wonderful and I will never forget that. The two girls were so excited about the care package they made me. It was so thoughtful and it was made with so much love.

In the midst of all this loving and caring, in the back of my mind, I was still angry. I was angry with the doctors who didn't care to do anything in the beginning of this nightmare. I couldn't erase this anger I had towards them. If they had done their jobs, I wouldn't be going through all of this pain and suffering, physically and emotionally. I know I made it this far through the love and care of my family and friends, and all those who cared and loved me. The doctor's before, I felt, ruined my life and my appearance. Why couldn't they have just listened and cared? Why couldn't they have just done their jobs?

I had to learn to overlook those feelings of hatred and try to focus on the present. I now had good surgeons, whom I trusted to make me well and whole again. Even though I will be scarred for life, they are doing what they are supposed to be doing. They are doing the right thing. They are healing me, and caring about how I feel, while at the same time doing a wonderful job.

When the surgery day finally arrived, I was so very scared. But as I do, I picked myself up, proud and strong, and did what I had to do. My mother taught me to be that way. Even though she lived in another state and could not be there for me, she was there in spirit, and I knew she was praying for me every minute.

It all seemed quite routine, and normal, waiting my turn for the surgery since I had been through all this before. I went on the usual road to the prep room, where you relinquish all your belongings to a plastic bag with the hospital's name on it. Which of course you get to keep when you go home. What a convenient thing to have. And oh, who doesn't love those gripper socks you get. What a treat. They are actually fun. I would make them in bright florescent colors though. The gowns are a little more comfortable and there are many nurses attending to your needs. There was the usual series of questions and note taking. All the time the other nurse at your side is trying to get your intravenous line into your arm. After all this is done, you get to take the glorious trip to the restroom. Why do they do that? Since I spoke before of the trials and tribulations of this whole ordeal of the restroom walk, I won't go into it now.

Once you are back into your bed, safe and sound, it is time for the anesthesiologist to come in and assure you it will all be calm and easy. But in my case, it makes me very ill, and also the fact that I am an asthmatic plays a big part in all this also. He informed me that special precautions will be taken in my case, and all would be fine. He eased my fears, and I knew everything would be fine.

And now comes the wait. You speak to your loved ones, or friends, and you assure them it will all be all right. Even though you yourself wonder. You wait for the time when you will go in, and for now you hold hands and give kisses. All the time, your heart is racing; waiting for the time they will take you into that cold room where your life will change forever.

And now you see a nurse come your way. It is your turn. Your heart beats fast. Everyone says their goodbyes and you quickly get whisked off down the corridor to the awaiting operating room with many nurses and professionals awaiting your arrival. It's your day to shine. Though me laying naked for a few dozen people isn't my idea of shining. Nevertheless, I watched everyone getting ready, and everyone hustling about. Everyone has something to get finished before the big moment.

You are slowly moved onto a table, which is cold as ice, I might add. It isn't easy to get comfortable on a rock hard table and being so cold you shake.

You have one person making sure you are straight. You have another person setting up your blood pressure machine. Then you have another person strapping your arms down. That is a feeling you remember. At that point in time, you know they are in control. You have people behind you, people on the side of you, and you have a nurse, far off in your view, opening up all the instruments that will be needed. I remember thinking, what an enormous amount of tools. Did they really need that many? The nurses were getting gauze and bowls ready, making sure machines were working properly, and the anesthesiologist near your head waiting his time to shine.

You really don't have too much time to think, you seem to be more into observing everything around you, than you have time to think about what is going to happen. I remember looking at the clock and seeing how wonderfully precise and on time they all were. That was comforting.

I remember some nurses asking questions, or just trying to hold a conversation to help ease the tension. They want to make sure that you are calm. They give you another blanket to keep warm but I doubt that it stays on very long. But at the time it feels comforting. At least you won't know when the time comes that they take it all off. By then you won't be feeling a thing. They come over and adjust the large overhead light, to just the right position and you know then, it's show time.

The doctors make their entrance and assure you with covered faces, that everything will be all right. They tell you that everything is going smoothly and on schedule, and it's time to relax, and let them take over. I knew that now it was time for them to do their job. A job it took them years and years to learn and perfect. I knew deep down in my heart that they were going to do a wonderful job. I was safe and secure in their hands. I was confident in my surgeons.

They usually warn you of the time when the anesthetic will take effect. I normally don't like the "count backwards" approach or whatever they like you to do. I usually just put my mind into a happy place. I put myself into a time or place where I was so calm and peaceful and content. Walking on the beach on a warm summer day with a light breeze was my special place to go. The feeling of sun on my body warming me, and the sand on my feet, and oh those wonderful sounds of the waves hitting the shore in a wonderful sort of song. I looked for that kind of peace and tranquility. That is the way I like the anesthetic to go into effect. It works wonders for me.

Well, now it's time to think about that happy place, and let the doctors work their magic. It was a time to put myself into their hands. It was the time to be trusting. It was the time to feel whole again. It had been a long road of discouragements and disappointments to lead up to this moment, but I will emerge a different looking person, but on the inside I will still be myself, and all that makes me be me.

CHAPTER 7   AWAKENING

I guess the time in surgery went quickly. I was told later that all went smooth as planned. My old cancerous breast was then dyed, marked, and put into separate cases as to the different sections removed. And then off it went to the pathologist. I was hoping they would do a good job at deciphering the contents. Incisions were done, and stitches were made to the plastic surgeon's satisfaction. All without me realizing a thing. It is truly amazing what they can do. You put all your dreams and hopes of the future into their hands.

I can barely remember awakening in the recovery room. I guess the anesthetic really did its job. I know while going in and out of sleep, that I wasn't throwing up. This is something that I normally would be doing if they didn't know ahead of time. That was all I cared about at the moment. I was so very relieved at that moment because I was afraid I would bust my incisions open if I got ill.

I must have still been under the powers of the anesthetic, because I don't remember being put into my room either. I remember feeling awake for the first time, when the tremendous pain was there. It was so excruciating. At this point I could not have the usual morphine, so a substitute was issued. Something milder had to be given. I cannot explain the feeling of going from being glad it was over to going into the horrendous pain. My lower abdomen had been cut from hipbone to hipbone. Since they took the muscle from the abdomen and brought it up from there thru my chest to my breast area, it made it very painful from my shoulder to the abdomen. A large binder or girdle as you might imagine was put around me, which covered a good portion of my mid section. It was as tight as they could get it. I remember calmness for a moment then sheer horrifying pain coming after. It was sort of like the feeling of labor, quiet then pain you couldn't control. I have no idea why it was happening that way but that is how it was for me. I had a very rough time during my recuperation my first two days in intensive care.

The days went by with me being taken very good are of in the intensive care unit. Nurses were very attentive to my bandages, tubes and drains. But that was about all they could do. The healing was up to me, and how I would handle it. I had a choice, to lay there in a stupor getting all the drugs I could or just face the pain and deal with it, and my will to recover. I did just that. I relied on my strong will to keep me partially awake and moving just a small motion to keep going. I also treasured the compassion and help of my family and friends.

After a day or two I was put into a regular room. It was kind of nice getting into a room that was nice and bright and quiet, not a nurse in every minute to check on you when you just wanted to sleep or just wanted a moment to myself. It was a good time to collect my thoughts and gather up my strength.

I wasn't very eager to move out of bed, but if I could, then the catheter would come out and that would be one less pain and one less bag to carry along.

The nurses, by the doctor's orders, try to get you up as soon as they can. It's much better for the healing process if you can get out of the bed and at least sit in a chair for a moment. But first, you must get out of the leg restraints that you are in. I guess they aren't really restraints, but they are material wraps that go around your lower legs. They are hooked up to a machine that sort of massages them periodically. It helps with the healing and I think helps prevent clots in your legs. They feel really funny when they are on, but they really do make your legs feel better when lying in a bed for so long.

As I waited for all this to happen, I finally took a peek under the sheet. And to my surprise, there wasn't a huge bandage on the breast. There was just a small bandage covering my new breast. My new beautiful breast the plastic surgeon had given me. It was hard to tell exactly what it looked like laying down, but at least I knew it was still pink and it was alive. That is very important circumstances when you have a tram flap done. It must stay alive with the blood flowing to keep it on.

Well, the time came for the nurses to do their convincing that I could get out of bed and it would be all right. I thought, "I have a girdle like contraption wrapped around me I can barely breathe and you want me to get out of bed"? But at this time, I knew it had to be done for my own good. So one nurse got the wonderful lifeline, the bag and the pole ready and the other took my leg cuffs off, and grabbed an arm to try to get me out of the bed. Oh my goodness, how hard that was. I couldn't really sit up on my own, so I literally had to be pulled up to a sitting position, all the time taking little short breaths. "I can do this", I thought to myself. I just kept repeating that statement to myself, "I can do this".

The nurses were very patient with me. They don't let you go far away from their grip. I managed with their help to stand up by the side of my bed. Finally, after days, I was in a vertical position. My head started to spin, but quickly got better with a few deep breaths. I was standing. My abdomen felt like someone was pulling it apart in two. Yes, standing was a difficult but it had to be done, and actually felt like it was such a great accomplishment. It was a start.

All this time, you had your lifeline and urine bag, and you also had what's called "the bulb", strapped to your thigh to catch the blood that was draining from a tube inserted in the side of your chest. You stand there with all of these wonderful belongings attached to you, and you try to walk. The first step seems like a child's first step. They were very small and so very unsure. You are so afraid you might fall. But you go on. You know you must. I gathered up all my strength to take those steps over to the awaiting nurse by the chair. It seemed like it took forever. She helped me slowly ease myself into the chair. It was very hard work but oh how glorious it felt to sit in a chair for a short time. You can actually enjoy just a little bit more of freedom to take control of your own life again. Life's little pleasures all come one at a time.

As you try to keep your composure, the nurses try to change the bedding as fast as they can. It does feel wonderful to have clean sheets on the bed. Their efforts were greatly appreciated at that moment. You watch as they effortlessly put everything back on the bed in precise order, as it should be. The pillows positioned just the right angels to get you back into bed easily. Now they are finally finished and you are starting to get tired easily.

Now you actually realize that you must stand up, walk back to get into bed. There is no easy way of accomplishing this endeavor.

The nurses each take an arm and help you back up into a standing position. You could never do this alone. It takes an enormous amount of strength and willpower to get into a standing position again. You walk back to the bed slowly, thinking, " how am I going to get back into bed". Being a short person, vertically challenged, as my stepson would say, the bed seemed so high even when the nurses lowered it. You learn to face away from the bed, hold onto the nurses and either try to sit and swing your leg on the bed or crawl them inch by inch until you are in a sitting position in the middle of the bed. This is not easy to accomplish. I think everyone who has had to do this takes a deep breath at this time and think, "it's almost done". At this time, the nurses put up the back of the bed so it's not so hard for you. All you can do at this point is take another deep breath and lean back until you touch the back of the bed. I remember my abdomen pull so hard it sent shock waves through my body.

Then comes the moment you don't think of, the changing of the bandages and the emptying of the bulb, that is attached to your side.

The bulb part was easy. They teach you to just lift the lid, and it empties into a measuring cup. This way each time you do it on your own, you know to write down the measurements. At the top of the bulb is a stopper. You just open the stopper squeeze what is inside out into the measuring cup. Then with all your strength you squeeze the bulb hold it that way and replace the stopper to create a suction which in turn makes the bulb fill up with excess fluid from the incision site. Not a nice thing to have to do but necessary.

The breast bandage wasn't bad at all. I have to have paper tape because I am allergic to regular tape. This paper tape comes off rather easily. I could now partially see the new breast from a sitting position. It looked wonderful. The new bandage was put on ever so gently. The nurses were wonderful.

Now it was time for them to lay you back and undo the binder that holds you in to change your abdominal bandages. I was thinking it would not be so bad. The nurses slowly lower the bed to a laying down position. This is painful but also necessary. The binder had held you in so tightly that it was a relief to have it off. But what you don't realize is when they take that binder off, your muscles tend to move in different directions once released, and that wasn't so pleasant. I couldn't see the incision at the time because of the position I was in, but I knew it was big. They tried to change it the best they could without hurting me. Now that that was done, it was time to put the binder back on. They pulled up very tightly from either side of my body and closed the binder once again. Though it was painful, it actually felt better to have it back on.

Now, finally with all this actually finished, it was time to rest. They did one more check of the machines, for heart rate, temperature and blood pressure and it was over.

Now this was truly enough excitement for one day. But little do you know you'll get up again for the same routine later in the day. After all, it's for your own good.

I must have dozed on and off all that day. The pain from the day before had seemed to subside little by little. I could move more in the bed and my head surely seemed a lot clearer.

That day, late afternoon, dinner was finally brought. For the first time, I actually wanted something to eat. They keep you on a light diet, but for me, it was fantastic. Enjoying every bite and oh, that cup of coffee I so wanted. I felt a lot better after that.

But unfortunately, you have to digest your food, and it subsequently means a trip to the restroom, which in fact is a long way off. This is a glorious moment to the nurses, but not so pleasant a trip for you.

So you get your buzzer, and ring for the nurse. They arrive to help you out of your confinement to move out of bed. They remove your leg wraps, unhook the machines, grab your urine bag and your lifeline, and you are ready. You recollect the procedure of getting out of bed from the last time, so you manage to repeat the procedure and get to your feet. With all of your belongings, you are helped to the restroom, which seems so far away. The nurses are very good about trying to help you in any way possible. You make it in the restroom and realize the door closes and you are alone. You are actually standing alone. Something you haven't done in a very long time. In a way this is good, in a way standing alone is very frightening. At this moment you realize that you have to figure out how you are going to go about sitting on "the throne" as some people call it. The best way to do this, I thought, was just take a deep breath and sit. When you are done, you are left with the problem of using the toilet tissue. Now you have to realize, at this point, you are still connected to the lifeline via an IV in your hand. The other hand is holding the metal bar so you don't fall. Ok, then you think, "What's the solution"? You let go of the metal bar and just do it. Then you realize you have to take another deep breath and try to stand. You finally get enough courage to do this task and you make your way to the door. Now stand the nurses, waiting to help. How wonderful it is to see them and how wonderful they are. They are like little angels. Painstakingly you make it back to bed with the help of your guiding angels.

Now, little do you know, now that you have accomplished this great feat, they will want to take the catheter out since you have proven you can make it to the restroom and back to bed. It is not a procedure that is a hard thing to do; you just dread it getting done. It's not that great to think about. You have to lie there while a nurse comes and pulls a tube right out of you. But quickly, the whole procedure is done, and the bag is gone. Actually, it is a good thing because there is one less thing to carry around with you. Now you can feel that you are in charge of yourself just a little bit more. Every little accomplishment means a lot at this stage of recuperation. You are still hooked up to your lifeline, your bulb, your machines, and your leg wraps, but I guess you can't ask for everything. This is wonderful in itself.

The evening goes by in and out of sleep, loved ones visit, and nurses still come in periodically to check on you and take your temperature and your blood pressure. Check your legs for swelling and find out if you need anything. But after all this has gone by, you finally rest and doze off into a quiet slumber you so much deserve at this time.

I awoke to a sunny morning. One I decided would guide my day. God gave me this sunny day to awaken to and if he chose to let the sun come up, so can I.

I got enough courage and strength to get myself un-hooked from my leg wraps, grab my lifeline and slowly move myself out of bed. It took longer than I thought it would and was a little more painful than I expected, but oh how proud I was of myself. I am sure if the nurses saw me at that moment they would be quite upset at this accomplishment, but it meant a lot to me.

I decided to do this little feat for a reason. I so wanted to walk over to the large mirror and see my body. See what they had done to it. I would be able to look at my new cancer free body. I could see my new shape and also my new scars. I was so curious that it gave me strength to get up and just give it a look. I am not sure if it was just curiosity but it worked.

I slowly made it to the mirror in my room. It wasn't far away from the foot of the bed so I figured I would be just fine. Balancing myself so I would be secure, I gently pulled down the shoulder of my gown to reveal my new breast. How glori-ous that moment was. I could finally see that everything was all right. I could see how perfect and round it was. And it was very pink and healthy looking. That moment eased my mind. The nipple area was left off to make sure the healing went well, and could be put on later. Can you imagine that? That surgery was hard for me to imagine. They take your own skin and make it into a nipple and surrounding areas are tattooed to make it match the other. How cool I thought. I didn't care if it wasn't there at the time it was still beautiful.

Then I decided to remove the binder. It was something I knew I really shouldn't do, but stubborn as I am I decided just to go ahead and do it. It was difficult to remove. It closes with very strong Velcro so it was hard to pull. I was truly shocked at what I saw when I took it off. I didn't expect the incision to be that big. It kind of gave me a sick feeling, but I was satisfied that it was done and the incision looked clean. I then pulled the binder as tight as I could and it was back in place.

Throughout my days in bed, I had been feeling a very sore spot on my back, kind of like a burning sensation. I could not in my wildest dreams figure out what this could be from as nothing was done in that area. I decided to open the gown and take a look as long as I still felt I could stand there. To my surprise, my whole back in the shape of a square was red like a burn. It really stung. I didn't know what it was or why it was there. I just decided I would ask the nurse later and show her.

I heard a man's voice from behind me say "good morning". It was my plastic surgeon. I got caught. He was surprised to see that I was up and around by myself. I guess he realized just how stubborn and curious I was. I asked him what the large red square on my back was. He said that since I was on the operating table for such a long time, the liquid they use to prep your skin for surgery seeped onto the table under me. My skin was so sensitive, that I made the mark from prolonged exposure to it. He wanted to see the breast and how it was healing. I opened my gown and he went to check the incisions. As I looked into the mirror, I was standing in front of, I new something was just a little different. As I looked, I noticed that there on my abdomen, was a different bellybutton. How strange. We all get to know throughout life what our bellybutton looks like. This one was not mine. I asked the plastic surgeon about it. I said to him "is this a new one". He said, "Yes, we had to make you a new one because the old one was cut off when we stretched your skin to where it is now". I was truly surprised and didn't expect that, but it was ok it was cute. And bellybuttons at my age really didn't mean a whole heck of a lot.

The plastic surgeon said that I was doing exceptionally well, and I could have my intravenous taken out but had to stay another day. I sure was happy to hear that comment. I thanked him especially for that one. I didn't mind staying another day if that was taken out. My surgeon left the room with a smile on his face.

Now the nurses stepped back into the room. It was time to take the intravenous out. How wonderful was the knowledge that it would one less thing to lug around with me. It was a little more freedom, one step at a time. What a long journey it was already. The procedure went smoothly thank goodness and the needle was gone. What a relief.

The evening went much smoother. All day I was able to get up and down, with only having to unhook my leg wraps. That wasn't an easy thing to do because you have to bend forward to do it and you have this large binder stopping you from bending. But if you have determination, everything is possible. I walked to the window during the day and I walked a little in the hallway that evening which was wonderful, being away from those same four walls I had been put in for days.

That night was a peaceful sleep finally. I slept soundly knowing I was getting much better and could be able to go home in the morning. A day I longed for.

I awoke in the morning refreshed and anxious for the surgeon to come in and say it was ok to leave. Time was going to slow for me. I wanted to be able to go home. I had some breakfast in the morning sun by my window. I knew this would be a good day because God saw it to give me another sunny day. I had a feeling this would be the day I could leave and go to my quietness and my loved ones and my dogs. They had been so lonely without me I imagined. I couldn't wait to show them some affection. And show them that everything is ok. They are like children. They need to be assured of things too.

If I were to be released, I would have to follow the nurse's instructions all the way. And there were many. The drain tube and bulb would not come out until a later surgeon's appointment. I had to promise to make sure I took all the measurements and keep them on paper. I knew I could handle that part if I went home. It would be a breeze.

Finally, the nurse came in and said, "The doctor will be here shortly". I knew he would let me go home. I knew I was doing rather well and that's what was so important to him.

He arrived with a cheerful "hello, ready to go home"? "You bet", I said in return. He said, "ok then, I will give the nurse the instructions and you can call for your ride". Oh what a wonderful feeling that was. Hearing those anxiously awaited words, finally. The hospital was very wonderful to me, but I had just wanted to be home and take my recovery day by day. I wanted to be able to depend on myself for what I needed once again. I had my new breast, my new outlook, and my new life cancer free. I thanked God at that moment because I knew everything was just fine.

OH MY GOODNESS IT HAPPENED TO ME

CHAPTER 8   RECOVERY

Now the time has come for you to go home. What a long awaited moment. You are filled with so much excitement. It's hard to contain yourself.

Now, the trip down to your car is an interesting one. They call for a wheelchair, which you must go down in. No walking allowed. Hospital rules. You sit in the wheelchair trying to balance your belongings on your lap, as they call someone to transport you down to your car.

Interesting enough it always seems like the person who shows up to take you down to your car, got their license at the Indianapolis 500. They arrive, take your chair handles, and off you go. I truly believe they should make wheelchairs equipped with seat belts for hospital transporters.

Once in the hallway, you get whisked down the corridor in a series of twists and turns to an awaiting elevator. At this point, your head is going through drastic equilibrium changes. You go from lying down in your bed for days, to sitting, to being whisked down the hall. Now, you have made it to the elevator. You slowly get backed into the elevator and they push the button to go down. I don't know about anyone else, but being in an elevator does summersaults in your stomach when you are healthy. Now, you are recuperating from pain medication, and you're being thrust down to a few floors below. At a high rate of speed I might add. I was never so glad to reach ground floor. It would be nice to be able to get off of that elevator. To be out of those four walls that surrounds you. I just wanted to see and feel the sun on my face again.

So now, you need to get out of that elevator. So they move you out, if you are lucky, you get someone who takes the first step slowly. And also you might get one that will inform you that there will be a small bump as you exit. But then again, you might have the qualifier for the Indianapolis 500 who just takes it like a bump on a dirt track.

Then you finally make it to freedom. The glass doors that hold you in are now opening to let you out. You manage with all your might to climb out of the wheelchair into your vehicle. You sit in your seat in your vehicle and realize, though very sore and very tired from the excursion, that you are going home, and you are free.

The ride home was that of holding a pillow on the front of my body to ease the bumps in the road. Once home, the healing was very tiring and painful. The breast area was healing well. The tube still inserted in my side to drain excess fluid from the surgery site was still draining steadily, but the abdomen was very sore.

I had to go through the usual daily process of emptying the bulb, and measuring it, and keeping a record of those measurements, by day and time and quantity. Since I was a person who had employment with financial records and used spreadsheets a lot, I just made a spreadsheet to keep track of all the numbers that needed to be kept. Doing it this way made it very easy to take these measurements to the plastic surgeon for my appointment.

The abdominal incision didn't do so well. It seemed to be always oozing and didn't look that good to me. It was very red all around the cut line. Then after a few days, the redness stretched out, but near the incision line it was a very funny color of skin. It was very pale. I was getting worried. I called the plastic surgeon's office and he wanted to see me right away. He sensed something was not right. So, like a good little soldier, I trudged along to the plastic surgeon's office, even though I just wanted to lie down and rest.

When I arrived, he slowly took the dressing off the wound. At that moment, a terrible look came across his face. I thought to myself, "do I look that bad"? I guess, as it turned out, the skin surrounding the incision site was dying. Yes, dying. I never heard of such a thing. I was shocked and I was scared. What now? My surgeon said they would have to repair the area. He had his office schedule an appointment to "fix the situation". Well, the appointment was sort of like a surgery day. They needed to go back to the incision site and cut out a section of skin all around the outside from hip to hip. It sounded awful to me bet had to be done. No choice at this point. A new incision line was made and closed and a tube inserted in the incision for drainage.

I returned home with not only a new incision to take care of, but also there was another drain. This one I had no bulb attached to, it just drained onto bandages. My days from then on went from taking care of the "bulb drain", and also taking care of the new drain. At times I got so frustrated with it all, but I knew it was for my own good. The more they drained, the better I would get and be a little bit closer to being normal again.

As days went by, I noticed that my abdomen started to get larger. Not from eating it was just getting so huge. I started to get worried because in that area above the belly button, there was no incision site. So, I wondered why it was so large. It wasn't hard, it was soft, like full of fluid and it was getting pretty sore. Another complication I thought. So I called the plastic surgeon's office. He said to come into the office and he would take care of it. I guess it was something that was "normal" in some people. I had to end up being that person. Of course, it isn't easy to drive yourself to the doctor's office with the incisions and the drains, but I did accomplish this feat with great results. I was proud of myself in fact. I did something on my own. It sort of proved to myself that I did have my freedom, limited, as it was I had it.

A wonderfully sympathetic nurse took me into the exam room, had me change into a gown, and await his arrival. Now being a normal person off the street, I had no clue as to what this swelling meant. It worried me. The minutes seemed endless until he arrived in the examination room. In he walked with his wonderful warm understanding smile. He said, "What seems to be the problem"? I went on to explain the swelling and how sore it was. He explained to me that it was just fluid build up from the surgery. Some people get it some people don't. I am one of the lucky ones to get it. He went on to say that it would have to be drained. I didn't want to hear that either. I had been through so much already. It seemed like that would be a procedure I wouldn't want done at this time, but knew I had to even though I was so sore. After all, he knew what was best for me so I let him know it was all right.

He explained that the nurse will be back in with the "necessary equipment", and we could take care of it.

The nurse came back into the room with packages and swabs and gauze. It didn't look good to me. I asked her "plain and simple, how is he going to do this"? She went on to explain that they'd clean off my abdomen to make sure it was sterile and the doctor will insert a needle and drain it out. At that moment, my heart sank. She said that it shouldn't be too bad because the pain nerves in the abdomen are not yet right from the surgery, so I shouldn't feel too much. I couldn't comprehend what he was about to do. I couldn't imagine what it would be like or what he would be taking out. I was worried at this point.

I thought it would be a needle and syringe like they use for shots. Oh my goodness was I wrong. When the nurse took out the "equipment", there was a large needle connected to a very large syringe, the size of a small cucumber. I never even knew they made them that big. Now I was really a bundle of nerves.

Then the moment I feared. The surgeon came back into the room. Normally, you await his arrival to come quickly, but this time I did not. I knew what was going to happen. I thought they would insert a small amount of numbing solution, but to my surprise, that didn't happen. They did just the cleaning off to be sterile. Before I knew it, the surgeon had placed the needle with the large syringe attached to it against my abdomen and just pushed it in. I think it took me by surprise, but there was really no pain. I couldn't believe it. As I watched him, I saw him pull the suction of the syringe up which made it fill up with a bloody liquid. I lay there afraid to move. I could not believe what was coming out of my abdomen. It actually filled to the top. I still was in shock and in wonder of it all. At that point, he pulled it out and then it was over. Then a small piece of cotton and a band aide were put on it and that was it. I was so glad that it was over. So then the surgeon turned to exit the exam room and he turned around and looked at me and said, "I will see you back in two days and we will drain it again". It was statement I couldn't believe that I was hearing. I guess at this point in time, it would be an ongoing adventure until the fluid build up would slowly ease up and eventually stop. This was not something I wanted to do or was prepared to do. Especially knowing that I would have to drive there and drive back afterwards. But it had to be done.

OH MY GOODNESS IT HAPPENED TO ME

As I drove home, it started to hurt. It started to sting really. I couldn't imagine doing this again. After all, I had a tube in the lower incision, a tube still in my side, and now this. I just couldn't believe that my body was reacting this way, but it was.

On my next visit to get drained, the plastic surgeon decided it was time to take the tube out of the hip-to-hip incision, as it really wasn't draining that much anymore. So I laid down on the table as I do when he does the syringe draining, and he removed the bandage to the incision with the drain. In a blink of an eye, he pulled the tube out. I guess it was the best way to get it done. It was the element of surprise. No time to think about what he was about to do. One less tube I have sticking out of by body. That was a very good feeling at the time. Then there was the taking of one more mega syringe of fluid out and it was time to go home. The drive was hard and exhausting, but I did make it home. Now, it was time to relax.

During this entire ordeal, I still had the drain tube in my side and the long tube connected to the bulb. I had been sleeping in my recliner because it was just easier for me to get up and down. I decided to get some rest and sat down in my recliner, nice and cuddly, surrounded by pillows wherever I could fit one in. I sat in a variable cloud of pillows. I rested, and it felt so good to just relax after the day's medical experiences. Resting was a good thing.

I remember this experience not for the fact that I rested, but for the fact that a dreadful occurrence happened after the little nap.

I decided to get up and get a drink of water. I slowly pulled the handle on the side of my recliner to bring my feet down. A procedure I did many times. I situated myself so I could easily stand up. I did. It was not a good thing.

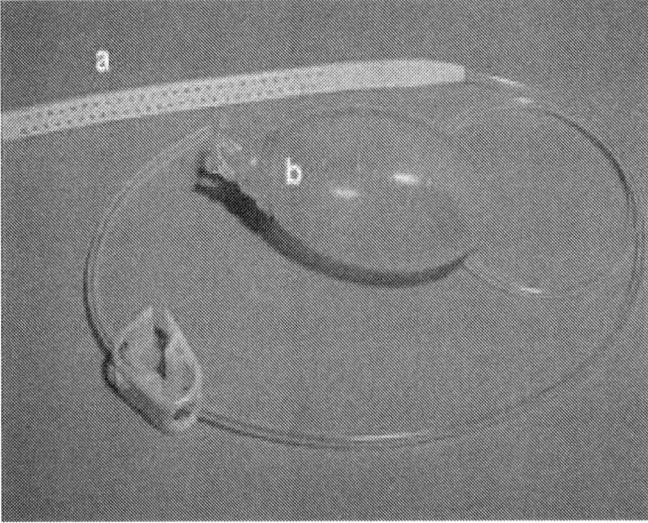

As I rose up from the recliner, I had unknowingly shut the recliner footrest on the tube and the bulb that was coming from my side of my breast. Now this tube is sewn with one stitch to your side, holding it to your skin. When I got up, it pulled the stitch out that held the tube in place to my skin. The stitch broke. Now, let me explain that the tube is not only inserted into your side, but there is another piece about the size of your little finger in width and length placed inside your body also. This little plastic piece has little holes in it, which makes the fluid go up into the tube, into the bulb. So, when I got up, it not only broke the stitch, but also pulled this piece of plastic half way out of my body, while the other half was still inside of my body. I was in total shock at this time. I was alone, and I knew I couldn't panic. I had to be in control. I never even knew this part was inside of me. No one had informed me of what was put in on that end.

At this point, I had to figure out how to sit back down in the recliner, all the time holding this piece that was protruding from my side. I had to manage to sit down, lean back holding everything, and pull the foot lever up so I could get the tubing out from in the chair. This was a really hard thing to do since I was in total shock and also had to hold my side tube so nothing else came out. I managed to get this feat accomplished and I stood up. By now my head was spinning from shear exhaustion and fear. I held all the pieces in and managed to get to the phone. I called the plastic surgeon's office but it had already closed for the day. I talked to a lady at the answering service for the doctor and she suggested I call the emergency room right away and see what they thought I should do.

So, I called the local emergency room, explained my situation, and they said that they would have a physician call me back shortly. Just to take it easy and try not to move. Easier said than done I thought. Here I was with a plastic contraptions sticking out of my side and I was supposed to just take it easy.

The minutes seemed like hours, while I waited for someone from the emergency room to call me back. Finally, the phone rang. It was one of the emergency room physicians. A polite sounding physician was on the phone ready to give me advice. This was a relief. He asked me about how far the plastic piece was sticking out of my side. I proceeded to tell him that it was half way out I thought. He said in these words, "Ok, now take hold of the piece that is closest to your body, and pull it out". I know I was in shock then. Pull it out? Reluctantly, I did what he wanted me to do. I had pulled it out of my body. To my surprise, it didn't hurt to badly. I sat there and looked at it then said to the physician, "what do I do now"? I think at this point, he knew I needed some relief from the stress and he said calmly, "throw it away". Well, that seemed like a good idea, but it wasn't exactly what I meant. There was still an open hole in my side where the piece of plastic was to deal with. I said to him "what about the hole"? He said to take a piece of gauze, and stick it in the hole and cover it with more gauze and call the plastic surgeon the next day. Then he said, "Have a nice day". I said "thank you and goodbye", and hung up the phone. I walked to the restroom and looking into the mirror, I was proud of myself for performing the task that was asked of me. No matter how crazy it seemed at the time, I did it. Now I had no more line or bulb attached to my body. Oh what a feeling that was. I didn't have to drag that thing around with me everywhere and no more draining and measuring. It was a good thing I thought in the end. But boy it had been a long day. But now, I could rest comfortable without that contraption. And I did.

The next day I called the plastic surgeon's office and told them of my experience. To say the least, I guess the way I explained it to the nurse, she had a good laugh. Now that it was over, I needed to have a good laugh too. She then talked to the plastic surgeon and he said just to come in the next day as usual for the draining unless something else came up. Heaven forbid anything else should happen I thought. This was more than enough for me. I guess he learned that when it came to me you might as well expect anything.

In the midst of all this commotion, I noticed that where he had just taken the drain out of my lower abdominal incision, the area was turning red, and there was like a pouch below it. I couldn't believe my eyes. Not something else I thought. By this time I was physically and mentally exhausted. I finally just had to lie down and get some rest and not think of anything that had to do with my body. I just wanted to be at peace.

Awakening in the morning, I felt a heavy feeling on my gauze that was on my abdominal incision. I looked at it and it was full of blood. I called the plastic surgeon's office again, and they said he was in the hospital doing rounds. They paged him and he said to tell me to meet him at the emergency room. What next I thought. I got my self together and like a trusting little soldier, I drove myself to the emergency room.

When I arrived there, they were expecting me. He had informed them that I would be coming in and to call him when I arrived. They took me to an examination room, had me lie in the bed and took the old bandage off the incision. My plastic surgeon arrived shortly thereafter. He took one look at it and said he suspected that it was infected and the amount of blood that came out was just a pocket that had formed from the fluid.

At this point I thought he would just put some antibiotic on it and some bandages. No, not with me, he reached beside himself on the counter and grabbed a large swab like cotton on the end of a stick. He proceeded to put this large swab deep inside the whole. At that moment, it really hurt. But he explained that that is what he would need to run the test for infection. At this time he prescribed an antibiotic for the infection that he suspected I had. I took the antibiotic as he told me to do, but ended up being allergic to it. I ended up with blisters inside of my mouth from it. Now on top of everything else, my mouth was in pain. I was so depressed at this point. This made the healing time even longer.

Now, the draining of the abdomen took place every three days. At this time, he would check that wound and make sure it was healing ok. Little by little it started to close but very slowly. It was important that this wound close, because as long as it was an open wound, my future treatments whether it be chemotherapy or something else, could not be started. It seemed to take weeks but it started to heal. I was surely glad of that. I was so tired of changing bandages.

Now that I was healing and the drainage amounts were less, I could actually see that I was getting a little bit closer to where I wanted to be health wise. I knew I had a very long road ahead of me, but if I could get through as much as I have gotten through already, the later part would be a breeze. I just need to have confidence in my physicians, and confidence in myself that I could do this. I could win this battle. This little soldier was mightier than anyone could imagine and I will beat this. I will win this war. I knew if I could get through all of this, everything would be just fine. So, I thought.

OH MY GOODNESS IT HAPPENED TO ME

CHAPTER 9   LEARNING THE FUTURE

As the weeks were going by, draining, and healing, I was set up to see an oncologist. We would be talking about future medical treatment options that we could take.

The oncologist was a young doctor, but very very knowledgeable. He tried to explain to me the best that he could what it was I could expect in the future as far as treatment goes. He didn't go into detail just yet, but he gave me brochures explaining the things that I would be going through, not just physically, but mentally. He spoke of how treatments would go, and how many I would possibly have. He did try to tell me everything that I would need to know.

He then decided to do an examination. I had to do the regular routine of putting on a gown while waiting for him to come back into the room. All the things he had mentioned to me were rushing through my head. I had never been around someone who had to have chemotherapy, so I really did not know exactly what to expect.

He entered the room and started the exam with my new breast. He said that the breast was healing beautifully and looked very healthy. Then he looked at the hip-to-hip incision. As soon as he saw the hole, he was not pleased. He said, "We can't start any of your treatments until this is healed up 100%".

I was devastated. I wanted to get the treatments he spoke about over and done with. I had already been prepared for the impending hair loss, loss of appetite, and fatigue. I just wanted to get it over with so I could go on and get myself back to at least a partially normal life again. I wanted a normal life like other people have. I didn't want a continuing saga of bandages, medications and treatments. That was what I was hoping for. Just to be what I considered normal.

At this point, the oncologist said that once it had healed completely to call his office and make another appointment to come in. At that time we would make arrangements to get the treatments started and get on a regular schedule.

I left feeling informed, yet in despair. He tried his best to comfort me before I left, but nothing could have prepared me for the extra time that had to be taken to let things heal.

My journeys to the plastic surgeon's office for draining continued. The only hard thing that there was now was the fact that now I would have to stand and get the abdomen drained. Yes, standing. It was the same procedure just in a different position. It was very hard. I had to stand with my arms out to my sides, and he would stick the needle with the syringe attached to it right into wherever he could feel the fluid buildup. Sometimes it would take a little turning or moving of the needle just to find the pocket of fluid. This was very hard to watch being done, let alone having it done. Not a comfortable feeling at all. But, he was a very compassionate surgeon through the whole ordeal. He knew I was scared. He knew how stressful it was on me, but we had to get it done.

Finally, through many draining visits, the hole in my abdominal incision started to completely close. What a wonderful relief that was. I was happy because now we could go on. But at the same time, I knew what was awaiting me in my future. I couldn't imagine the weeks of chemotherapy I was going to have to receive. How would I handle the new look of being bald? Would I be too fatigued to be able to work at my present employment? Being a Personal Assistant to an Entrepreneur, there were many people I would have to deal with in the course of my employment. Many of them I saw on a daily basis. Could I do it in my present condition? I would spend many days at meetings with realtors, designers, bankers, builders, and captain of the yacht and crew. It was a very busy occupation, but one I truly enjoyed doing. I wondered if I would be able to handle it all as usual. Would the way I look change how the people I dealt with see me? Will they be able to work with me like they did before? All these questions came into my mind. Will I be able to hold up the energetic life I was used to doing? I wondered if the chemotherapy would hinder my clear thinking which was so very important to my occupation. All these things made me aware that my future was in question. My life was going to take a big turn and I will be expected to go on as normal. I needed my wits about me. I knew I had to get myself together, not only physically but most of all mentally to continue as before. I needed to do whatever it took.

My employer was very understanding during this whole ordeal. He knew all that I was going through, minus the medical details of course. He so kind-heartedly bought me a computer system for my home and sent all his files to my home also. File cabinets installed, desk installed, extra phone lines, whatever it took to make my life easier was done. Being able to work from home during this time was just wonderful and truly a blessing. I would still meet with people, outside my home, but most of my monetary work and secretarial work I could do there in the comfort of my surroundings. It made life so much easier for me. It truly was wonderful. It made me feel just a little more confident that I could get this done and continue as I did before which meant so very much to me.

Through all the pain and suffering, and through all the worries, and fears, I was alive and life was good. It truly is taking a turn for the better. My outlook was better and that in turn made me feel better. I think your attitude at a time like this is very important. You must keep up. You must hold your head up high and say that this can be done no matter what.

I was so glad that I could continue my job with hardly any obstacles to stand in my way. No hair? Oh, wigs and bandanas work wonders. Tired? Just go take a nap. If there was so much work to be done? Take a break. There were ways of handling anything that would come my way. And I did. I wasn't going to give up.

CHAPTER 10 REACHING THE END OF THE JOURNEY

The weeks of healing went by and for once I was feeling good. The pain was easing, and the incisions were healing. Now that these things were happening, it brought about the reality that more was to come. The days of chemotherapy were drawing nearer. At this stage, the chemotherapy would be all right I thought. I've been through so much that it had to be all right. I would make it seem just fine.

I knew the expectation of loosing my hair, and feeling tired, and the feeling of not wanting to eat a thing, but nothing prepared me for the new problems that I would be having.

The oncologist made the date as to when I would receive my first chemotherapy treatment. Now that that was made, I started to get scared and my mind started to wander. I wondered how would I react? Will it be easy for me or hard on me? At this point deep inside, I wondered could I do this.

I arrived at my appointment like a wide-eyed child. As usual, the nurses were very polite and wonderful to me and tried to make me as comfortable as possible mentally. As the time approached, we walked down a hallway to the room where I would be for my first treatment. I wondered what it would look like. What kind of things would it have in it? Would it be as beautiful as the rest of the facility or a depressing room?

As I walked into the room, I could see a row of recliners. Yes, recliners. In most of the recliners there were people hooked up to bags of dripping medication. Some were with their family members, some alone. Some were reading, some were sleeping, and some were just talking with their loved ones or friends.

The nurse told me to go ahead and choose a chair. As I surveyed the room, I saw a recliner that was by a large window. I decided that would be the best place for me. I loved the outdoors, so I figured I could lie there and look outside until my treatment was over. So, I walked over to my recliner and got comfortable. They offered blankets and pillows. They tried to make me as comfortable as they could in the chair. It's a nice feeling when you know the hospital workers really care how you feel. They know and realize how worried and scared you are at this time. I sat in my recliner actually very comfortable watching the other patients. They also seemed comfortable and at ease. That was good.

I noticed the nurse coming towards me with a rolling tray. We all know the steel one on casters that bring the "equipment" to you. There were needles and more gauze and a syringe. Oh, and let us not forget the metal pole that is just like the ones that hold your lifeline in the hospital. Things were going well. I looked at all the things that were going to be hooked up to me as I sat. Then I noticed those wonderful plastic pans they give to patients when they get nauseous. Now, just the thought of seeing that pan sitting there sent a little sign of getting worried that I might need it at some point in time. I didn't like that feeling. I had to calm myself down and regain my composure. The nurse informed me that she would be putting a needle into my arm so the medication can be administered. It was just like the lifeline. It was just another intravenous hookup that we all know and love.

They informed me that the doctor would be close by just in case I get a bad reaction. Now that was something to tell someone, before they get the medication. I know it made me worry more. But I guess they have to inform you of these situations and how they will handle them if they occur. I guess it is better than the element of surprise.

The first dose of medication was from a bag at the end of the metal pole. I was told at this point that if I felt nauseous from the medication they could give me a pill. That statement made me feel so much better. I truly hated the thought of getting ill at that moment and how awful it would be. I hated to be sick in front of all the other patients, maybe my being ill would make them ill and I would feel just awful.

Now they start the medication. They really do try to make you feel as comfortable as possible. Blankets are offered, pillows are right there for you so you can rest comfortably in the recliner. And usually there are plenty of magazines to read if you like. It all was made to be very comforting surroundings. And of course, I chose the chair by the window so the warm sun was on my face. What a gift from God that was.

As I lay there letting the cure run through my veins, I remembered something a friend told be before I went for the chemotherapy appointment. She said, "always picture your chemo medication as knights in shining armor going through your body slaying all that was bad inside you with their trusty swords". And I did just that. I closed my eyes, rested, and envisioned the battle.

After a time, in that chair, I started to get fidgety, lying in the same position. I decided to sit up and look out the large window I was seated next to. It was a beautiful, warm, sunny, day. How wonderful the sun felt warming my face and body as it shown through the window. It felt so wonderful. But then everything changed.

As I sat there, I slowly started to feel funny. My stomach started to do summersaults, and I knew what would be happening next. I tried not to think about it but there was no ignoring this feeling of illness. I summoned one of the nurses and subsequently used the plastic pan that they had provided for people like me who just couldn't manage the chemotherapy. She summoned one of the other nurses to get me the pill that would control this awful feeling. I took it with great willingness. A short time after that they informed me that they would be giving me another form of chemotherapy, but it would be in a syringe and administered by hand by one of the nurses. The chemotherapy would have to be put in at a very slow rate straight into my arm. I did not expect that.

As I sat waiting for this other chemotherapy drug, I envisioned a small needle and syringe like they give shots with.

I knew that at this point, they would give me the syringe of medication and I could go home. Along came a nurse with the equipment needed for this last procedure. To my surprise, lying there on the steel wheeled table was a syringe the size of the one they used to use to drain my abdomen. This syringe was filled with a bright red liquid. The nurse sat down next to my chair with all the equipment ready. He inserted the syringe into my arm and slowly, very slowly, started to inject this red liquid. I only remember that it felt cold going inside of my body. The nurse was very pleasant the whole time but it was a strange experience for me to handle at the time. I couldn't wait for him to get the syringe finished and take it out. But I knew I had to just wait and let the nurse do it slowly.

Now as this was going on, I had that feeling of impending illness fall over me again. Luckily, there was a new plastic pan close by. It was not their fault that it affected me that way, but they did show their concern and said they were sorry it had happened that way. They decided to make me stay just a little while longer until the feeling passed. All the medication that I was going to get for that day was over but I needed to get over this feeling I had now. It got easier but it didn't pass.

I was worried because I had to drive myself home. I had to get myself together. In the process of getting ready, the nurses were informed that I did have a previous Medical Assisting Degree. They made it much easier because they would call a pharmacy and have them give me a syringe filled prescription to take home and administer to myself to stop the nausea. I agreed.

I drove myself to the neighborhood pharmacy. My feeling of illness subsided to a small extent. I had that wonderful extra paper bag we always manage to have in our vehicles from the last fast food restaurant we visited still stashed away in the car. I walked through the pharmacy talking to myself into not being sick here in the store.

I handed the prescription to the pharmacist and went to sit and wait in the waiting room. To my surprise they called my name rather quickly. I was so happy to be able to go home soon. I walked over to the pick up window and the pharmacist said, "We don't carry this kind of medication and we don't have enough syringes to fill it". I was devastated. My stomach did another turn. I explained to them that I had just had my chemotherapy treatment and was feeling pretty ill. I asked them if they could please call around for me to other pharmacies. They politely said they would but it would take a little time. I went and sat back down in the waiting room and waited. I watched as customer after customer went along their way. I just wanted to be home and resting. Finally, they called my name.

I went to the window and the pharmacist said they found one pharmacy that had enough vials and syringes to fill the prescription. What wonderful news this was for me. I asked where the pharmacy was, and it turned out that the pharmacy was across town and had no delivery service to offer. I thanked them politely and went to my car for my next driving adventure.

The drive wasn't too bad. I found the pharmacy fine and the prescription was waiting for me. I thanked God for this one little favor.

By this time I was so worn out. I drove myself home. I think as soon as I got home, and greeted my loving dogs, and fed my fish, I gave myself my first shot and decided to lie down. How wonderful it felt being in my own home, in my own bed, and having my dog at my feet taking care of me. She always did.

I had two weeks in between treatments, so I had time to recuperate and get back to work. How I enjoyed this time, because it actually gave me a chance to feel just a little normal again.

It seems like your life is split into two ways of living when you go through all of this. Your life is with doctor's appointments and nurses and tests and medications. And then there is your other life, of trying to keep up with family and friends. The other half of your time is spent trying to figure out how to get the grocery shopping done, house cleaning and clothes washing done while you feel so tired you just want to rest. But you naturally figure things out and do the best you can. There is always tomorrow.

As I sat daily, trying to think of all that needed to be done, not only at home, but also, for my employment, my wonderful lab decided that she had to go outside. As she nudged my leg to get my attention, as she normally does, I noticed something on my lap. As I went to brush it off, I realized it was my hair. I was warned that it would start falling out, but I guess I never noticed it before. I had short hair at the time so it really wasn't noticeable to me. I let my labs outside, and decided to go look in the mirror. At this moment I don't know why, but my heart was beating fast. I knew what to expect but just didn't want to face it. I looked into the mirror and saw a patch of my hair missing. I don't know why, but I decided to brush my hair. As I took the brush through my hair, the hair came out in the brush and fell to the sink. I just burst into tears. I couldn't control them. I guess it was all that had been before stored up inside and had to be let out. There I was, standing in my little pink bathroom crying uncontrollably. I went to my bed, leaving the brush in the sink and just cried some more. I cried myself to sleep.

I then awoke to hear my dogs wanting back in the house. My lab knew something was wrong. She could just sense it. She gave me extra loving that day. She knew.

The next day I decided I had better get a grip on things. I decided to go buy some bandanas. They were the easiest thing for me do put on my head without hair. There were so many different patterns of bandanas; it wasn't so bad after all. I even found one with dollar bills printed on it I decided I would wear for my meetings with financial people. In a way it was just a fun thing to do to make the situation just a little more comfortable.

The weeks went by and the more hair I lost and the more treatments I received, the more anger built up inside of me because I did not receive the treatment I should have had in the beginning. I knew I had to put it all behind me, and try to move on, but it hurt and it left a permanent mark on my heart and soul.

Finally, as the sun shown in the sky, the day arrived for my last and final chemotherapy treatment. It was the day I had been praying for. It was the day I had so long awaited. It would be no more days of medicines and injections. I could be normal again. The day it would all be over.

I could now go on with my life. I had to realize it would be a life of taking a pill every day for the next five years, but I could handle that compared to all I had been through. It was a very long, hard journey. It was a journey that I would remember vividly for the rest of my life. Many lessons were learned from this experience. I learned to just take one day at a time and enjoy each day to it's fullest no matter what happens.

I decided to walk the beach along the ocean that day. I felt the sun on my face, and listened to the sound of the waves hitting the shore. I felt the sand between my toes and just thanked God I was alive to enjoy another day with my family and friends and pets, and live more of my life. I was so happy at that moment. My life was returned to me. Yes, it would be a different sort of life. But it was a life I was given to live and that I will.

A SHORT PEEK AT BOOK II

OH MY GOODNESS IT HAPPENED TO ME

BOOK II

THE JOURNEY OF REOCCURANCE

OH MY GOODNESS IT HAPPENED TO ME

Days went by, and months went by with the glorious feeling of being healthy. I finally started to enjoy life once again. Every day seemed like a blessing. I had not only one but numerous days that I could enjoy the wonders of our world. Each day I awoke with the knowledge that I was able to get up do the normal things people did every day. Something that was taken away from me long ago when I discovered I had cancer.

Those days seem like a dream now. The pain, the suffering the agony the embarrassment and the shame were over. And the agony of being embarrassed that I was different was over. The feeling that I couldn't have a life like everyone else because of my illness. It really is an odd thing how illness will play with your emotions. I still to this day haven't gotten my strong will back. But I will in time. It seems that illness can break the even strongest of will. The harder the illness the weaker your will is to fight. It seems easier to give up than to fight the fight. Many days were filled with just that. But somehow, the human soul survives and the will gets stronger and the fight gets easier and the days get brighter with every minute. And you learn to take advantage of every wonderful moment in time. That is what is important now. The thought you put far back in your mind is, that you don't have to go every day thinking, "what if it comes back"? You don't want to even think of that happening, but the possibility is always there. It will always be there. You don't know when or you don't even know that it will, but the possibility is always there. You just have to learn to live your life without that thought. You go on with your everyday lives, go to your appointments as scheduled and hope that the day will never come when you hear those words "the cancer has come back".

www.ingramcontent.com/pod-product-compliance
Lightning Source LLC
Chambersburg PA
CBHW031216270326
41931CB00006B/576